Don't Touch My Prostate!

A Man's Guide To Curing Prostate Cancer — No Scalpels, Radiation or Side Effects!

by Lee Euler
With Susan Clark

'Don't Touch My Prostate!'
A Man's Guide to Curing Prostate Cancer — No Scalpels, Radiation or Side Effects!

By Lee Euler

With Susan Clark

Published by Online Publishing & Marketing, LLC

A Publication from *Cancer Defeated*

IMPORTANT CAUTION:

By reading this special report you are demonstrating an interest in maintaining good and vigorous health. This report suggests ways you can do that, but — as with anything in medicine — there are no guarantees. You must check with private, professional medical advisors to assess whether the suggestions in this report are appropriate for you. And please note, the contents of this report may be considered controversial by the medical community at large. The authors, editors and publishers of this report are not doctors or professional health caregivers. The information in this report is not meant to replace the attention or advice of physicians or other healthcare professionals. Nothing contained in this report is meant to constitute personal medical advice for any particular individual. Every reader who wishes to begin any dietary, drug, exercise or other lifestyle changes intended to treat a specific disease or health condition should first get the advice of a qualified health care professional, or accept full responsibility if he or she decides not to do that.

No alternative OR mainstream cancer treatment can boast a one hundred percent record of success. Far from it. There is ALWAYS some risk involved in any cancer treatment. The authors, editors, and publishers of this report are not responsible for any adverse effects or results from the use of any of the suggestions, preparations or procedures described in this report. As with any medical treatment, results of the treatments described in this report will vary from one person to another.

PLEASE DO NOT USE THIS REPORT IF YOU ARE NOT WILLING TO ASSUME THE RISK.

The authors report here the results of a vast array of treatments and research as well as the personal experiences of individual patients, healthcare professionals and caregivers. In most cases the authors were not present themselves to witness the events described but relied in good faith on the accounts of the people who were.

ISBN 978-1-4507-4113-2

© Copyright 2010 by Online Publishing & Marketing, LLC, P.O. Box 1076, Lexington, VA 24450

All rights reserved. No part of this publication may be reproduced, stored in a retrieval system, or transmitted in any form or by any means, electronic, mechanical, photocopying, recording or otherwise, without the prior written permission of the copyright owner.

Printed in the United States of America

About the Authors

Lee Euler has written about alternative health for 17 years. His books and articles have been read by millions. He's written for publications edited by Dr. David Williams, Dr. Julian Whitaker, Dr. William Campbell Douglass, Dr. Mark Stengler, Health Sciences Institute and others. He's the editor and publisher of several reports on alternative cancer treatments, including *German Cancer Breakthrough* by Andrew Scholberg, *Cancer Breakthrough USA* by Frank Cousineau with Andrew Scholberg, and *Natural Cancer Remedies That Work* by Dr. Morton Walker.

Susan Clark is a freelance writer who has spent the last ten years writing about health and nutrition. She's written for publications edited by Dr. Jonathan Wright, Dr. Julian Whitaker, Dr. David Steenblock, Dr. Al Sears, and many others. Before that, she spent nearly a decade researching health news and current events for leading news organizations across the country including KTLA-TV in Los Angeles where she won 3 Golden Mic awards, and her work was nominated for an Emmy.

Table Of Contents

Chapter One
Prostate Cancer: To Treat Or Not to Treat?
The Surprising Facts about "Watchful Waiting"..page 1

Chapter Two
Prostate Cancer Treatment No. 1
Dr. Douglas Brodie's Immune-Boosting Therapy ....page 5

Chapter Three
Prostate Cancer Treatment No. 2
Advanced Prostate Cancer Disappears with a "Japanese Secret" for Long Life!
The Healing Power of Macrobiotics... page 13

Chapter Four
Prostate Cancer Treatment No. 3
The Amazing Non-Toxic Liquid that Killed Virtually 100% of Cancer Cells
Within 48 Hours at the National Cancer Institute!.. page 18

Chapter Five
Prostate Cancer Treatment No. 4
Flood Your Body with Oxygen and Cancer Cells Will Die On Contact:
The Budwig Protocol.. page 22

Chapter Six
Prostate Cancer Treatment No. 5
Cutting-Edge Sound Treatment Melts Away Early Prostate Cancer!
High-Intensity Focused Ultrasound — HIFU.. page 26

Chapter Seven
Early Detection of Prostate Cancer
The Problem with PSAs and the Test That's Working Better .... page 32

Chapter Eight
Diagnosing Prostate Cancer
The Biggest Problem with "the Gold Standard"— Ultrasound and Biopsy .... page 37

Chapter Nine
The Hidden Dangers of Conventional Prostate Cancer Treatments
The Truth about Prostatectomy, Radiation and Hormone Therapy… .... page 41

Chapter Ten
Why So Much Prostate and Breast Cancer?
The Truth about a "Hidden" Epidemic! .... page 47

Chapter One

Prostate Cancer: To Treat Or Not to Treat?

The Surprising Facts about "Watchful Waiting"

There's a saying that doctors around the world have repeated for decades: *If you live long enough, you'll get cancer.* It's not a pleasant thought, but it's true. And surprisingly, it's even *truer* for MEN than for *women!*

Researchers estimate that prostate cancer will attack <u>ONE OUT OF EVERY SIX MEN.</u> And the disease strikes far *earlier* than you'd ever imagine.

Researchers now believe up to *20 percent* of men over 50 already have prostate cancer. And the older you get, the greater your danger. By age 70, the number of men with prostate cancer DOUBLES to *40 percent*, and by 85, it soars to *60 percent!*[1]

It's a scary thought, isn't it? Well, don't worry just yet.

You can live your whole life with prostate cancer — many men do!

Though prostate cancer can be very serious, it's far from a death sentence. Prostate cancer is *unique* among cancers. Unlike breast, colon, lung or even brain cancer, it's RARELY detected during one's life — at least, historically speaking, before the current mania for cancer tests.

You see, many men with prostate cancer live out full, active lives with the disease and then die of *something else altogether!* In fact, a wealth of research suggests many men today have *"microscopic"* amounts of cancer in their prostates and don't even know it. That's because the cancer never grows enough to be a real problem.[2]

For example, in a study published in the journal *Age and Ageing,* coroners autopsied men of all ages who died from causes *other* than cancer.

When they examined the men's prostates, they found cancer cells in ALMOST ALL OF THEM. But the cancer was so small it didn't cause any real problems for the men's health. In fact, most of them probably didn't even know they *had* prostate cancer![3]

The truth about treating early prostate cancer

Now, please don't misunderstand me: I'm not saying prostate cancer is *"no big deal."* Prostate cancer is a terrible disease that takes many different forms. And in its most aggressive form, prostate cancer can quickly drain the life out of you, like a vampire in a horror movie.

But the point I want to make is that as medical technology becomes more precise and as earlier detection of prostate cancer becomes possible, men need to be clear on a very important medical truth:

---

1 Harwood, Rowan. Review: Should we screen for prostate cancer? *Oxford Journals. Age and Ageing.* 1994. 23. 164-168.

2 Harwood, Rowan. Review: Should we screen for prostate cancer? *Oxford Journals. Age and Ageing.* 1994. 23. 164-168.

3 Harwood, Rowan. Review: Should we screen for prostate cancer? *Oxford Journals. Age and Ageing.* 1994. 23. 164-168.

Being diagnosed with early prostate cancer might not be as serious as many conventional doctors believe.

Early prostate cancer doesn't necessarily warrant aggressive treatment - or ANY treatment at all, as far as that goes. The facts have clearly shown that the disease can take so long to develop that for many men it'll never pose a serious threat to their health.

Getting NO treatment is "__BETTER__" than chemo, radiation or even surgery!

Dr. Willet Whitmore, the father of urologic oncology, was one of the first to make this discovery. He's well-known for saying, *"For a patient with prostate cancer, if treatment for cure is necessary, is it possible? If possible, is it necessary?"*

When it comes to conventional treatment for prostate cancer, a wealth of research suggests that the answer to Dr. Whitmore's question is a solid *"no."*

In a shocking 1992 study of 223 prostate cancer patients, researchers found that *getting no treatment* was actually BETTER than any standard chemotherapy, radiation or surgical procedure! The results were so groundbreaking, they were published in the mainstream *Journal of the American Medical Association*.[4] Later, a second alarming study reported similar results.

85 percent lived longer by *refusing* conventional treatment!

In this second study, wrote researchers in the *Journal of the National Cancer Institute*, men who received no treatment for their prostate cancer survived at an 81 PERCENT HIGHER RATE than those who underwent radiation therapy.

And those untreated men survived at an 85 PERCENT HIGHER RATE than those who got hormones or submitted to castration for their tumors.[5]

That's right, men who had no treatment at all for their prostate cancer LIVED LONGER than those who received standard, conventional treatments!

But *"no treatment"* doesn't mean going about your daily business and pretending you don't have prostate cancer. You see, in these studies, patients used a virtually forgotten technique called *"watchful waiting."*

"Watchful waiting"...what does it mean, exactly?

Watchful waiting is the *regular monitoring* of your prostate tumor to see whether it's growing, and, if so, how quickly. Doctors and patients use this information to determine whether your tumor will threaten your health or will never be a problem.

Though "watchful waiting" clearly is effective for many men, conventional medicine rarely recommends it.

An article in the *Journal of the American Geriatrics Society* said more than 90 percent of all doctors who recommend surgery NEVER tell their patients that watchful waiting is an option.[6]

Why? In many cases the reason is *money*.

Cancer is an *industry*. And "watchful waiting" makes no money for conventional doctors or their hospitals. In fact, doctors and hospitals probably fear they could LOSE MONEY if a "watchful waiting" patient went on to get prostate cancer, then filed a malpractice lawsuit against them.

---

4   Johansson JE, Adami HO, Andersson SO, Bergström R, Holmberg L, Krusemo UB. High 10-year survival rate in patients with early, untreated prostatic cancer. *JAMA*. 1992 Apr 22-29;267(16):2191-6.

5   Newschaffer, Craig J., et al. Causes of death in elderly prostate cancer patients and in a comparison nonprostate cancer cohort. *Journal of the National Cancer Institute*, Vol. 92, April 19, 2000, pp. 613- 21

6   Fowler FJ Jr. Prostate conditions, treatment decisions, and patient preferences. *J Am Geriatr Soc*. 1995 Sep;43(9):1058-60. No abstract available.

So it's no wonder that doctors are grossly overtreating many prostate cancer patients with risky treatments for tumors that might never put the patients' health or their lives in any real danger!

Many of these doctors may believe they're doing the right thing – heaven knows why, given the evidence to the contrary – but it's a plain fact that the "right thing" as they see it lines their pockets with cash.

More than one million men are being dangerously "overtreated" for prostate cancer!

A study published in September, 2009, in the *Journal of the National Cancer Institute* shows just how bad the prostate cancer overtreatment problem has become.[7]

The study revealed that routine "prostate-specific antigen" (PSA) screening for prostate cancer has caused more than *one million American men* to be diagnosed with a prostate tumor and get treatment for it, when it might never have caused them a single problem!

A recent online Health Alert from Newsmax.com quotes the lead author of the study, Dr. H. Gilbert Welch, as saying, *"These are men who could not be helped by treatment because their cancer was not destined to cause them symptoms or death."*[8]

You have up to a 49 in 50 chance of being *overtreated*!

Dr. Peter Bach of Sloan-Kettering told the *New York Times* that if a man has a PSA test today, *"It leads to a biopsy that reveals he has prostate cancer, and he is treated for it. There is a one in 50 chance that, in 2019 or later, he will be spared death from a cancer that would otherwise have killed him. And there is a 49 in 50 chance that he will have been treated unnecessarily for a cancer that was never a threat to his life."*[9]

But what makes this cycle of overtreatment even more upsetting is that conventional prostate cancer treatment breaks the Number One law of medicine: *Do no harm.*

Tragically, countless men are suffering the pain and terrible discomfort of surgery, the long-term dangers of radiation treatment, and the loss of precious quality of life — not to mention the emotional stress and the financial costs!

Conventional treatments are taking men's prostates and leaving them with *bladder problems, erectile dysfunction* and *bowel urgency*. In many cases, they're WORSE OFF *after* treatment than they were *before*!

Safe alternatives for treating early *and* advanced prostate cancers

The alarming research that's being published today is why I believe that getting the word out about *safe, alternative treatments* for prostate cancer is more important today than ever before in medical history.

Let's face it, when you KNOW you have cancer in your prostate, you want to get it out. And *fast*. Even if "watchful waiting" is a valid choice for you, it won't help your peace of mind to know you have cancer slowly growing in your prostate!

But now, while you "watchfully wait" to see whether your tumor will grow and become a threat, you can also start taking very simple steps to *cure* the cancer on your own, with no horrible risks. I'll show you how in the next few chapters. And that's not all…

Should the worst happen and your tumor starts growing swiftly, or your cancer is already

---

[7] Welch HG, Albertsen PC. Prostate cancer diagnosis and treatment after the introduction of prostate-specific antigen screening: 1986-2005. *J Natl Cancer Inst.* 2009 Oct 7;101(19):1325-9. Epub 2009 Aug 31.

[8] "Prostate Screening: More Harm Than Good?" NewsMax Health. 2009.

[9] Kolata, Gina (2009) "Review of prostate cancer screening, Prostate Test Found to Save Few Lives" *The New York Times*

advanced, you'll also discover some extremely powerful alternatives that can help you get rid of your cancer without surgery, radiation or, God forbid, *castration*.

The dismal reality facing breast and prostate cancer patients today in conventional medicine is what inspired me to write this Special Report, because someone *must* tell you that treating prostate cancer doesn't have to be this way! In many cases, men can keep their prostates!

That's right, prostate cancer *can* be cured safely, permanently and without needless suffering and disfigurement — even after conventional doctors have given up all hope!

On the coming pages you'll discover lifesaving alternative treatments. Best of all, you'll see that their success is based not just on anecdotal evidence but on years of clinical use and scientific study.

In some cases, the alternative treatments you'll discover have undergone rigorously controlled, FDA-approved clinical studies that the government never releases to *you or the news media!*

In other words, these alternative treatments are the real deal. They can give you and your loved ones hope not only for survival, but for a healthy, high-quality life after cancer! After all, isn't that what it's all about?

Tragically, for most Americans, finding out about these exceptional alternative treatments has been extremely difficult.

Why you won't hear about these alternatives from your doctor

Even the most well-intentioned doctor *won't* tell you about these amazing treatments that are stopping, slowing and even curing prostate cancer. In fact, he or she *can't* tell you about them!

Why? Because the federal Food and Drug Administration (FDA) *forbids* conventional doctors to use "alternatives" to treat cancer. Your state's medical board can yank your doctor's license if they find out he or she has been breaking "the rules." Your doctor can even *go to jail* for prescribing what he or she believes is the best treatment, and several brave doctors have actually done so.

So when it comes to finding the best alternative treatment for your cancer, *you're on your own.*

Fortunately, several excellent books on alternative cancer treatments are available. But even they fail to tell you *which* treatments are highly successful against prostate cancer, in both the early and the advanced stages.

That's why I've compiled this Special Report: As a guide to help anyone who's facing prostate cancer.

In the pages ahead, you'll discover some of the leading-edge alternative treatments with high success rates in curing prostate cancer. And I'll tell you *exactly* where to get these treatments and use them, on your own or with expert help. That includes giving you the names and contact information of the alternative doctors who treat prostate cancer patients.

So let's get started!

IMPORTANT: Please note that I don't profit in any way from the treatments outlined in this Report. Nor do I have any financial connection whatever to the doctors on whom I report. After spending 17 years writing about health issues and finding out that alternative treatments cure countless people of prostate cancer, from early stage to "hopeless" stage-four cancers, I wanted to write this Report to get the life-saving information into your hands.

Chapter Two

Prostate Cancer Treatment No. 1

Dr. Douglas Brodie's Immune-Boosting Therapy

Peter R. was 67 when his doctor told him he had prostate cancer so advanced it would do no good to operate. Peter's PSA level was 17 TIMES HIGHER than normal — a frightening 71.4 (under 4 is considered "normal").

Stunned, the former police detective got a second, a third and even a *fourth* opinion. One doctor said he might live three years. Another told him he could "cut off his testicles" to try and stop the cancer's advance. But all four doctors agreed that Peter's prostate cancer was terminal.

"*They wanted to bury me,*" Peter later told Sacramento news reporter Melinda Welsh.[10] But instead of getting ready for the end, Peter used his detective skills to gather information on *alternative treatments* and interview prostate cancer patients who'd tried them.

He learned about an amazing clinic in Reno, Nevada, where a doctor named Douglas Brodie was curing cancer WITHOUT surgery, radiation or chemotherapy. And for the first time, Peter felt there was *real* hope.

Peter's PSA nose-dived to 00.1!

One month later Peter was on Dr. Brodie's natural anti-cancer program. His hopelessly high PSA began to drop, slowly at first, and then it *plummeted.*

Eighteen months later, Peter's PSA had dropped an *astounding 70 points* to a healthy 1.0. His "terminal" prostate cancer had VANISHED! And his recovery was no fluke. Two years later — and five years since his diagnosis — Peter is *still* healthy as a horse, and his PSA is a stable 00.1.

So what is Dr. Brodie's secret? *The immune system.*

Dr. Brodie, like many other alternative cancer pioneers, believes cancer develops in your body because *your immune system is weak.*

During more than 30 years of fighting cancer, he discovered a dozen natural compounds that work together to *power up* your immune system to SAFELY KILL PROSTATE CANCER — and many other cancers, including breast cancer.

Dr. Brodie's immune-building prostate cancer protocol

Dr. Brodie treated prostate cancer patients such as Peter with a daily IV (intravenous) infusion of powerful *antioxidant nutrients, minerals, enzymes, glandulars* and other *natural compounds* to repair their immune systems and fight the cancers. Peter spent two weeks at Dr. Brodie's facility, the Reno Integrative Medical Clinic, undergoing *daily* immune-strengthening infusions such as these.

---

10 Welsh, Melinda (2002) "Forbidden Medicine Cancer patients from Sacramento are seeking an alternative, holistic approach to building up the body and beating cancer. Too bad it's outlawed in California." California: NewsReview.com

While there, Peter also learned how to eat the *right foods* and avoid the *wrong foods*. Dr. Brodie put him on a diet HIGH in vegetables that are rich in beneficial *phytochemicals*. These phytochemicals build your immune system and fight cancer. These vegetables included *broccoli, cabbage, cauliflower and Brussels sprouts*.

When Peter got home, he also started taking a "home-care" regimen of *oral vitamins and supplements*.

Detoxify your body with colon hydrotherapy

Dr. Brodie also uses detoxification techniques to cleanse away immune-sapping toxins that have built up in his patients' systems over the years. His method of choice is *colon hydrotherapy*, in which a professional hydrotherapist cleanses the patient's colon with water.

"I have found over the years that cancer patients who are not doing well usually are toxic and not being cleansed. They certainly are in need of colon hydrotherapy," Dr. Brodie revealed in Dr. Morton Walker's article, "Value of Colon Hydrotherapy Verified by Medical Professionals Prescribing It."

"I do recommend that most of my cancer patients take colon hydrotherapy or 'colonic irrigations,' because they often improve by having such treatment. Liver cancer in particular shows benefit from colon hydrotherapy, but any internal tumors show effectual change, too," Dr. Brodie added. *"It's better than an enema, which is merely a lower bowel cleanse, as opposed to a colonic, which is a thorough cleanse of the entire bowel."*[11]

Relieves BPH and prostatitis, too!

Colon hydrotherapy helps men in other ways as well: It can relieve prostate enlargement, called benign prostatic hyperplasia (BPH), and prostate infection, known as prostatitis. Both are very common in men over 50.

The late Emil Sayegh, M.D., got wonderful results using colon hydrotherapy with men suffering from BPH or prostatitis. For more than 15 years he reported how colon hydrotherapy could solve frequent and painful urination in his male patients. When Dr. Walker interviewed Dr. Sayegh for his article on hydrotherapy, he explained:

"Cleaning the colon markedly assists the functioning of the pathological male bladder and prostate organs. Colon hydrotherapy given to involved men at two-week intervals for three times to start and then maintained every four weeks for an unlimited period does solve prostatitis and benign prostatic hyperplasia. From my files, I can offer up several hundred case studies which testify to that fact."[12]

Learn to control the "cancer personality"

Dr. Brodie also arms his cancer patients with valuable *stress-relieving techniques*.

"Most people who develop cancer are susceptible to stress," reported Dr. Brodie at the annual Cancer Control Society Convention in Pasadena, California, in 1992. Dr. Brodie described what he calls the *"cancer personality."*

"I believe that cancer begins from long-standing abuse of the psyche. By and large, cancer patients exhibit very similar conflicts, and these give rise to a well-defined cancer personality," said Dr. Brodie in a 2002 issue of *The Townsend Letter for Doctors and Patients.*[13]

The characteristics of this "cancer personality"

---

11 Walker, Morton D.P.M. (2000) "Value of Colon Hydrotherapy Verified by Medical Professionals Prescribing It," *Townsend Letter for Doctors and Patients.*

12 Walker, Morton D.P.M. (2000) "Value of Colon Hydrotherapy Verified by Medical Professionals Prescribing It," *Townsend Letter for Doctors and Patients.*

13 Walker, Morton D.P.M. (2002) "Profile of the holistic cancer therapist W. Douglas Brodie, M.D., H.M.D — Medical Journalist Report of Innovative Biologics," *Townsend Letter for Doctors and Patients.*

include being a "worrier." And someone who often puts other people's needs before themselves — "people pleasers," they're often called. These people are also dutiful, responsible, hard-working and usually of above-average intelligence. They often internalize emotions and hold on to feelings of anger or resentment.

In fact, Dr. Brodie says the link between cancer and emotional stress is so strong that he's seen the onset of detectable cancer in many patients two years after a traumatic life event.[14] But there's good news. You can cope with the cancer personality by altering your behavior and "reclaiming your power of healing". Dr. Brodie recommends:

- Eliminating "toxic" negative emotions and replacing them with positive ones
- Having faith in God or a higher power
- Relieving yourself of too many obligations and responsibilities — reduce your stress
- Being open and honest. Talk with others about the problems, conflicts or burdens you may feel[15]

By doing each of these things, advocates believe you're taking back control from stress and negative emotions and eliminating their dangerous power over your health.

The connection between a person's mental state and cancer is another area that remains controversial. I'm sure plenty of people who are happy and fulfilled get cancer anyway. I don't believe happiness or a positive attitude will cure cancer all by themselves, and I'm sure Dr. Brodie never said such a thing. Attitude is one part of a multi-pronged program to defeat cancer. Why not be happy and positive?

14 Walker, Morton D.P.M. (2002) "Profile of the holistic cancer therapist W. Douglas Brodie, M.D., H.M.D — Medical Journalist Report of Innovative Biologics," *Townsend Letter for Doctors and Patients.*

15 Walker, Morton D.P.M. (2002) "Profile of the holistic cancer therapist W. Douglas Brodie, M.D., H.M.D — Medical Journalist Report of Innovative Biologics," *Townsend Letter for Doctors and Patients.*

I can tell you this much: there's very good evidence that stress and depression damage your immune system and as we've seen, your immune system is your most important weapon against cancer.

Intravenous (IV) infusions and insulin-potentiated hypoglycemic therapy (IPHT)

One of the most important elements of Dr. Brodie's immune-boosting protocol is the daily intravenous infusions of powerful antioxidant *nutrients, minerals, enzymes, glandulars* and other *natural compounds.* These infusions can include:

- the powerful antioxidant vitamins A and C
- minerals such as potassium and magnesium
- digestive enzymes and CoQ10
- glandular supplements such as thymus (from the thymus gland)
- shark cartilage
- germanium
- Laetrile

Of course, each of these supplements is available at your local health food store (except for Laetrile). But please note: Taking the supplements orally may help your immune function, but they WILL NOT kill all of your prostate cancer.

Why? Because these supplements' effects on your immune system are only powerful enough to kill cancer when you take them *intravenously*.

When you do that, they bypass your digestive tract and go straight into your bloodstream, enhancing their effects. And they become MORE POWERFUL still when Dr. Brodie infuses *sugar* into the supplement solution.

The cancer-killing secret of sugar — yes, sugar!

Cancer cells love to eat sugar. And that's an important reason why Dr. Brodie's treatment is *so effective* against even "terminal" prostate cancer.

"The cancer cells open their membranes in response to a metabolic need for sugar as food by the insulin's producing a drop in blood sugar," explained Dr. Brodie to Dr. Morton Walker in The Townsend Letter for Doctors in 2002. As the cancer cell opens itself to "suck up" larger amounts of food, it also sucks up *"healing substances which cancer cells don't like."* This therapy is called insulin-potentiated hypoglycemic therapy or (IPHT).[16]

IPHT does to untouchable prostate cancer cells what kryptonite does to Superman-it makes them weak and virtually powerless. In layman's terms, here's how IPHT works: You're injected with insulin, which opens up "insulin receptors" or sugar receptors that cover cancer cells. When these receptors are open, cancer cells are automatically hungry for more sugar.

After you're given this insulin, you're fed sugar along with cancer fighting antioxidants and compounds. Cancer cells absorb the sugar and cancer fighters like drought stricken land absorbs water in a rain shower.

From the reports I've seen, IPHT can dramatically increase the strength of virtually any cancer treatment — natural or conventional. It works by getting more of the cancer fighting drug or natural compound into cancer cells.

Vietnam vet's "terminal" prostate cancer disappears

Like thousands of young Americans, John S.[17] was exposed to high levels of the toxic jungle defoliant Agent Orange while serving in Vietnam. Years after surviving his tour of duty, John watched seven men from his platoon die of cancer probably caused by Agent Orange.

In 2002, he thought it was his turn.

Doctors told him a biopsy of his prostate had confirmed that cancer was growing out of control. The results showed 10 OUT OF THE 12 TISSUE SAMPLES WERE CANCEROUS.

"I was advised that even with surgery and radiation, I would need a miracle to survive," John recalls.

Fortunately, he heard about the Reno Integrative Medical Center. John went for a consultation and decided to try Dr. Brodie's immune-boosting anti-cancer protocol. After 18 months, the tumor in John's prostate was *shrinking*. Four years later he's healthy, with *NO SYMPTOMS* of prostate cancer!

Dr. Brodie charged with criminal felonies for saving lives!

The natural compounds such as *shark cartilage*, *Laetrile* and *germanium* that are part of Dr. Brodie's protocol are being used in clinics elsewhere in the world to defeat cancer. But when doctors in the USA use them, they often face criminal prosecution. And Dr. Brodie is no exception.

On *three* separate occasions, government officials in California targeted him. And in the 1970s, the Board of Medical Quality Assurance charged him with 23 felonies.[18]

What were these felony charges for? Turns out they were for alleged "over-prescriptions" of

---

16 Walker, Morton D.P.M. (2002) "Profile of the holistic cancer therapist W. Douglas Brodie, M.D., H.M.D — Medical Journalist Report of Innovative Biologics," *Townsend Letter for Doctors and Patients*.

17 John, Case Study, Reno Integrative Medical Center, www.renointegrativemedicalcenter.com

18 Welsh, Melinda (2002) "Forbidden Medicine Cancer patients from Sacramento are seeking an alternative, holistic approach to building up the body and beating cancer. Too bad it's outlawed in California." California: NewsReview.com

prescription drugs. This included painkillers for a young man who suffered excruciating pain after having both legs amputated at the hip and both arms amputated at the forearm due to Buerger's disease.

"It was widely known that these attacks on my license were because of my use of Laetrile and [my] unorthodox approach to the treatment of cancer," Dr. Brodie explained to Sacramento news reporter Melinda Welsh.[19]

In fact, Dr. Brodie learned they were going to arrest him from reading about it in the newspaper!

Imagine opening up your daily newspaper and finding out you're going to be *arrested!* That's exactly what happened to Dr. Brodie! He had no idea they were coming after him till he read an article in the paper saying he'd been criminally charged — even though he'd been served with NO WARRANT or any other notification!

Later, in court, the medical board admitted it had erred in calling Dr. Brodie's prescriptions *"felonies."* The court *fully exonerated* him that time, and he was cleared again when they came after him a couple of years later.

But when California authorities sought to charge Dr. Brodie a THIRD time, he knew they'd keep hounding him with trumped-up charges as long as he kept practicing alternative medicine. In the late 1970s, he moved his clinic to Nevada, which lets doctors practice *some forms of alternative medicine.*

Not surprisingly, a short time later the state of California made it a felony for a physician to treat cancer with anything other than chemotherapy, radiation and surgery!

Laws such as these are one reason many conventional doctors shun alternative treatments.

---

19 Welsh, Melinda (2002) "Forbidden Medicine Cancer patients from Sacramento are seeking an alternative, holistic approach to building up the body and beating cancer. Too bad it's outlawed in California." California: NewsReview.com

Ask a conventional doctor about Laetrile, shark cartilage and germanium and he or she will call these treatments "shams" and the doctors who use them "quacks."

But clearly, they haven't looked at the research.

Laetrile study: 55 percent of TERMINAL cancer patients are still alive and well!

Case studies from doctors who use Laetrile (or *amygdalin*, as it's sometimes called), show this natural compound is MOST EFFECTIVE against cancers of the *prostate, breast, lung, liver and brain*, and *lymphoma*. Many of these doctors say Laetrile gives their patients a *better* chance of survival. Clinical studies back them up.

One of the most *impressive* studies was done by P.E. Binzel, M.D.

For 17 years, Dr. Binzel followed 108 cancer patients with metastatic cancer (cancer that has spread, and usually has a poor prognosis).

In the study's 17th year, 61 patients — MORE THAN HALF — were still alive. And *nearly half of those* had survived 5 to 18 years and counting after taking Laetrile as part of a nutritional cancer-fighting program.

These numbers are amazing. Even more amazing, nearly all these patients had *already been failed* by surgery, radiation or chemo. When they entered Dr. Binzel's practice, all were expected to die, yet an incredible 55 PERCENT SURVIVED![20]

Contains powerful cancer-fighting B vitamins

The scientific research also suggests *why* Laetrile is a powerful cancer fighter. Studies show it contains powerful cancer-fighting *nitrilosides* (vitamin B-17). Laetrile itself is completely

---

20 Binzel, P.E., (1994) *Alive and Well.* California: American Media

natural and is found in several nuts and seeds, including apricot seeds.

Interestingly, doctors studying primitive tribes in Africa, South America, Australia and other places found that their diets were FULL of nitriloside-rich foods. Many of these doctors, including the legendary Albert Schweitzer, M.D., theorized that their diets were a key reason there were no recorded cancers among these populations.

In Dr. Schweitzer's preface to A. Berglas's book *Cancer: Cause and Cure*, he wrote:

"On my arrival in Gabon [Africa] in 1913, I was astonished to encounter no cases of cancer. I saw none among the natives two hundred miles from the coast...."[21] The native diet was filled with millet and grains rich in nitrilosides.

Incredibly, the National Institutes of Health and the FDA *insist* that Laetrile does NOTHING to help cancer patients and is actually dangerous.

Cancer-fighting Laetrile "banned" by the FDA as a "poison"

The FDA banned Laetrile in the 1980s after allegations that the natural cyanide inside Laetrile could poison patients.

Does Uncle Sam have solid research to back this up? *No.* In fact, repeated studies in both animals and humans have shown that when used properly, Laetrile is COMPLETELY NON-TOXIC and free of side effects. Half a dozen alternative doctors, including Dr. Brodie, have reported no toxicity after using Laetrile with their cancer patients for decades.

Ironically, a conventional medical doctor who sought to prove Laetrile dangerous ended up providing more evidence for its high degree of safety. In his 1981 study published in the *Journal of the American Medical Association*, Dr. Charles Moertal wrote:

"In our study, intravenous amygdalin was found to be free of clinical toxicity and no cyanide could be detected in the blood... In summation, the administration of amygdalin according to the dosages and schedules we employed seems to be free of significant side effects. This conclusion appears to be validated by early observations in phase II study of 44 Mayo Clinic patients receiving intravenous amygdalin therapy and 37 receiving oral therapy who have not experienced any symptomatic toxic reaction."[22] [Emphasis added]

But even Dr. Moertal's own research wasn't enough to overcome his anti-Laetrile bias. He concluded the report with the statement: *"A definite hazard of cyanide toxic reaction must be assumed..."*

Well, you know what people say when you "assume" something? You make an "a-s-s" out of "u" and "m-e"!

The point is, research shows Laetrile is both *safe* and *very effective* when used correctly. But as cancer expert and radio commentator Bill Henderson often tells the cancer patients he coaches, Laetrile is not "a do-it-yourself operation." You should use it ONLY under a qualified doctor's supervision.

Study shows shark cartilage fights "terminal" cancer — results ignored!

Researchers have done several medical studies and hundreds of case studies on shark cartilage, but the most amazing research comes from William Lane, Ph.D., the founder of Lane Labs.

In the wonderful book *Cancer-Free*, Bill Henderson tells the incredible story of Dr. Lane and Charles Simone, M.D. These two doctors conducted a study that used shark cartilage on 29 "non-responsive" terminal cancer patients in Cuba in 1992.[23]

---

21 Berglas, A. Caassn (1957) *Cause and Cure.* Paris: Pasteur Institute.

22 Moertal, C. et al. (1981) A pharmacologic and toxicological study of Amygdalin *JAMA* 245:591-94.

23 Henderson, Bill (2008) *Cancer-Free (Third Edition)* Booklocker, Inc.

Five of these patients had prostate cancer, six had breast cancer, and the remaining 18 had other cancers. But ALL 29 had failed to respond to ANY conventional treatment. They were bedridden and expected to die within months. But after treatment with shark cartilage, an astounding 48 PERCENT – NEARLY HALF – *were alive and well almost three years later.*

As Bill Henderson reported in his book, Drs. Simone and Lane concluded that the shark cartilage stimulated the "*rapid growth of fibrin tissue (healthy tissue) replacing and encapsulating the cancer cells.*"[24]

As Dr. Lane recounted in a 1995 article in *Alternative & Complementary Therapies — A Bimonthly Publication for Health Care Practitioners,* although news media outlets such as "60 Minutes" with Mike Wallace were interested in the story, "*The National Institutes of Health (NIH), on the other hand, surprisingly, never took the time to hear the whole presentation, see the slides, talk to me, or talk to the interested doctors.*"[25]

Germanium: The natural "interferon" right under Big Pharma's nose

Germanium is a trace mineral that some healers have used since the 1960s to treat cancer and other degenerative diseases by enhancing people's immune systems. Specifically, it boosts the all-important tumor-fighting compound called *interferon* and your *natural killer cells.*

Ironically, Big Pharma has been trying to create drugs that boost your interferon for decades now, but they're always laden with dangerous side effects. Meanwhile, safe germanium has been available the *entire time!*

According to a study published in the *Journal of Interferon Research* and quoted in the book *Alternatives in Cancer Therapy* by Dr. Ross Pelton, "*Organic germanium restores the normal function of T-cells, B-lymphocytes, natural killer-cell activity, and the numbers of antibody-forming cells... Organic germanium has unique physiological activities without any significant side effects.*"[26]

Dr. Pelton also reports on *two* separate studies that show organic germanium stimulates the production of gamma-interferon in both animals and humans with no side effects or toxicity.

Plus, a number of human cancer trials, mainly in Japan, have found that organic germanium IMPROVED SURVIVAL TIME in several kinds of cancers.

In one study, patients' immune response and general health improved — even AFTER they received chemotherapy and/or radiation. Remember, chemo and radiation DESTROY your immune function, but with germanium, the patients' immune systems stayed strong!

This is worth repeating: You can use germanium WITH conventional cancer treatment to improve your immune system. This can help ANYONE with cancer!

It's also curing breast, colon, even lung cancer!

Besides working very well in advanced or aggressive prostate cancers, Dr. Brodie's immune-boosting therapy is also successfully treating three other kinds of cancers. Patients report being COMPLETELY CURED of colon, kidney and breast cancers. You can read many testimonials from former patients on the Reno Integrative Medical Center's Web site listed at the end of this chapter.

The most astonishing testimonial is from a man named Joe who was diagnosed with lung cancer — a cancer that's particularly hard to treat

---

24   Henderson, Bill (2008) *Cancer-Free (Third Edition)* Booklocker, Inc.

25   Henderson, Bill (2008) *Cancer-Free (Third Edition)* Booklocker, Inc.

26   Pelton, Ross, R.Ph. Overholser, Lee (1994) *Alternatives in Cancer Therapy.* New York: Fireside.

with conventional medicine.

After Joe underwent immune-boosting therapy at the clinic, his lung cancer *disappeared!* Joe writes:

"Today, I am free of cancer, without the trauma of chemotherapy or radiation. My energy and stamina have returned to that of a 40-year-old man, (not bad for a 71-year-old!)" [27]

Of course, conventional medicine continues to dismiss these recoveries as "spontaneous remissions." But Dr. Brodie knows better.

"My main objective over the past two decades has been to find those natural substances that most effectively enhance the immune system in its battle against cancer," he said in Dr. Morton Walker's book, *Natural Cancer Remedies*. *"When these substances are part of a comprehensive cancer treatment plan...the chances of beating cancer are markedly improved."*[28]

In 2005, sadly, Dr. Brodie passed away at 80 from a blood infection. But his clinic continues to treat cancer patients using the Brodie immune-boosting protocol, under the leadership of Robert Eslinger, D.O., H.M.D.

Dr. Eslinger has been in clinical practice for over 30 years. In November, 2008, Governor Jim Gibbons of Nevada appointed him to the state's Board of Homeopathic Medical Examiners.

For more information:

Reno Integrative Medical Center
6110 Plumas Street, Suite B
Reno, NV 89519
Tel: 775-829-1009
Toll-free phone: 800-994-1009
Fax: 775-829-9330
E-mail: rimcstaff@gmail.com
Web site: www.renointegrativemedicalcenter.com

To find a certified colon hydrotherapist near you, contact:

International Association for Colon Hydrotherapy
Post Office Box 461285
San Antonio, TX 78246-1285
Tel: 210-366-2888
Fax: 210-366-2999
E-mail IACT at homeoffice@i-act.org
Web site: http://www.i-act.org/IACTSearch.HTM

---

[27] Joe, Case Study, Reno Integrative Medical Center, www.renointegrativemedicalcenter.com

[28] Walker, Morton D.P.M. (2005) *Natural Cancer Remedies That Work Wonders*. California: Finn Communications.

Chapter Three

Prostate Cancer Treatment No. 2

Advanced Prostate Cancer Disappears with a "Japanese Secret" for Long Life!

The Healing Power of Macrobiotics

Dr. Tony Sattilaro was an anesthesiologist and the President of Methodist Hospital in Philadelphia. During a routine chest X-ray, the technician discovered a mass in Tony's chest. It was cancer. More biopsies were done. Doctors found cancer in his sternum, skull and spine, before they finally found the source of it: *his prostate*.[29]

Tony was shocked. He was *only 46!* It seems he'd fallen victim to an aggressive form of prostate cancer that strikes younger men. It had spread throughout his body, and now doctors were saying NOTHING could be done to save him.

Tony's prostate cancer kept spreading

Within weeks, the cancer invaded new bones and Tony was doubled over with pain. He needed narcotic painkillers just to get through the day. To make matters worse, his father was losing his own battle against lung cancer. And soon, Tony received the tragic news that his father had died.

His father's death was a turning point for Tony, but not in the way you might expect.

As Neal Barnard recalls in his book *Foods that Fight Pain*, Tony was driving back to Philadelphia after his father's funeral when he saw two young men hitchhiking along the highway. He needed the company, so he decided to pick them up.

How hitchhikers saved Tony with a "Japanese Secret" for long life

Tony told the hitchhikers his sad story, but they offered him no sympathy at all! Instead, they told him bluntly that his cancer DID NOT have to be a death sentence! By following an old Japanese eating secret for long life, they said, he could make the *prostate cancer go away*.

Of course, Tony didn't believe a word of what these two young hippies were saying. After all, he was a *doctor*! But he listened anyway.

The two went on and on about how food can heal your body by *restoring a healthy balance of energy*. They told him they'd learned WHICH foods can heal you at a school for *macrobiotic cooking*. Then they asked him for his address so they could send him everything he needed to know. The doctor in Tony couldn't resist, thinking "I've got to see this," so he agreed.

A couple of weeks had passed when Tony received a book on macrobiotic eating. Intrigued by a doctor's endorsement he found inside, he went to a local macrobiotic center and began eating the diet himself.

---

[29] Barnard, Neal D. (1998) *Foods That Fight Pain: Revolutionary New Strategies for Maximum Pain Relief.* New York: Random House

Three weeks later, Tony's excruciating bone pain was gone!

In just 21 days, Tony was feeling so much better that he threw away his painkillers. With renewed conviction, he continued the diet. Soon his energy returned and he felt healthier than he had in a long time. He kept waiting for the other shoe to drop, but it never did.

One year later, Tony returned to his doctor for a bone scan. The results were astonishing: There was NO SIGN of cancer in his skull, his sternum, his spine, his prostate or ANYWHERE ELSE IN HIS BODY!

Nearly 10 years later, Tony was STILL cancer-free. He'd left Philadelphia for Florida, where he spent his time writing about the relationship between food and health. He even wrote about his own experience in the book *Recalled by Life: The Story of My Recovery from Cancer*.

What is *macrobiotics*?

The word "macrobiotic" is a Greek word that means "long life." The macrobiotic diet was developed in the 1920s by George Ohsawa, a Japanese philosopher who taught that *simplicity* in diet was the key to good health. Ohsawa believed that by eating certain foods and avoiding others, you could cure yourself of cancer and many other serious illnesses.[30]

The macrobiotic diet resembles a *traditional Asian diet*. It consists mainly of *whole grains* and *vegetables*. For instance, on a macrobiotic diet you'll eat Miso soup, brown rice, lentils, and "sea vegetables" such as nori and kelp. Sugar, fat, meat and dairy products are off limits.

Today's best-known macrobiotic proponent is Michio Kushi. He pioneered the tailoring of Ohsawa's diet to meet individual needs, depending on age, gender, activity level, health and environment.[31]

In the article "The Macrobiotic Diet As Treatment for Cancer: Review of the Evidence," Joellyn Horowitz, M.D., and Mitsuo Tomita, M.D., break down the modern macrobiotic eating plan into food groups:

- whole cereal grains (40-60 percent of diet), including brown rice, barley, millet, oats, wheat, corn, rye and buckwheat; and other less-common grains and products made from them, such as noodles, bread and pasta
- vegetables (20-30 percent of diet), including smaller amounts of raw or pickled vegetables — preferably locally grown and prepared in a variety of ways
- beans (5-10 percent of diet), such as azuki, chickpeas or lentils; other bean products, such as tofu, tempeh or natto
- regular consumption of sea vegetables, such as nori, wakame, kombu, and hiziki — cooked either with beans or as separate dishes
- foods such as fruit, white fish, seeds and nuts — to be eaten a few times per week or less often.

How long do I stay on this eating plan?

Drs. Horowitz and Tomita note that for people with cancer, the macrobiotic dietary restrictions might be absolute for a period of time, till some recovery has occurred.

They also recount several case studies in which people avoided ALL animal foods and fruit, then reintroduced them to their diet. Again, it depends on your situation.

Interestingly, many macrobiotic "counselors" who help people use the eating plan to fight a variety of illnesses — including cancer — believe

---

30 American Cancer Society, www.cancer.org

31 Horowitz, Joellyn M.D., Tomita, Mitsuo, M.D. (2002) The Macrobiotic Diet as Treatment for Cancer: Review of the Evidence. *Complementary and Alternative Medicine*: Vol. 6, No. 4.

some people must stay on it *permanently*.

For example, in his book *Foods that Fight Pain*, Neal Barnard suggests that Dr. Tony Sattilaro's decision to stop eating macrobiotically caused his cancer to return, which then caused his death in 1989. Barnard writes, *"I would not see why he would want to do this [stop the macrobiotic diet]. A cancer that has been effectively suppressed is not the same as a cancer that is totally gone."*[32]

Clearly, Barnard believes the macrobiotic diet is not a *cure* but a *suppressive therapy*. And many doctors who use nutrition — whether macrobiotics or other diets — in their fight against cancer, believe the patient must ALWAYS stay with elements of the diet in order to maintain complete remission. Others might disagree.

Tulane University study: Advanced prostate cancer patients live THREE TIMES LONGER!

A graduate student at Tulane University did a study to see how well the macrobiotic eating plan healed prostate cancer. He examined the records of nine patients who'd seen a macrobiotic counselor for prostate cancer between 1980 and 1984.

He was shocked to discover that advanced prostate cancer patients who followed a macrobiotic diet survived THREE TIMES LONGER. The men who ate macrobiotically lived an incredible *19 years — nearly two decades* — compared to only six years for men who didn't follow the diet.[33] That's an extra *13 years* in which these men were able to enjoy their lives and their loved ones. And just as important, there were absolutely no side effects to damage their quality of life.

The Tulane student also found similar results in pancreatic cancer patients. The macrobiotic group survived FOUR TIMES LONGER than the control group.

But conventional researchers were quick to point out that the Tulane research didn't take place in a truly controlled environment. They say "other factors" might've influenced survival in both groups of cancer patients. Regardless, there are many reports of the macrobiotic diet healing cancer of *several different kinds* — especially prostate cancer.

The Prostate Cancer Research Institute and Dr. Mark Scholz published the case study of Thomas Mueller, a 45-year-old Los Angeles attorney. After being diagnosed with prostate cancer, Thomas refused surgery and all of the side effect-laden treatments his conventional doctors prescribed. Instead, he tried a *macrobiotic diet* and *exercise*. In just three months, his PSA had dropped from 4.0 to 1.5 ng/ml.[34]

"A-Team" TV actor free of prostate cancer 30 years later!

Do you remember actor Dirk Benedict from the TV show "The A-Team?" He played Templeton "Faceman" Peck, the suave, well-dressed member of the team.

When Dirk was in his early 30s and at the height of his career, doctors diagnosed him as having an aggressive form of prostate cancer. As he recalls in his book, *Confessions of a Kamikaze Cowboy*, doctors wanted to castrate him — imagine that happening to "Faceman!" *Not likely.* Well, Dirk thought the exact same thing. But what else could he do?

Fortunately, he was a close friend of the famous actress Gloria Swanson. Besides being a Hollywood beauty, she was a legendary proponent of the macrobiotic eating plan. Gloria told Dirk to go "macrobiotic" and to quit eating

---

[32] Barnard, Neal D. (1998) *Foods That Fight Pain: Revolutionary New Strategies for Maximum Pain Relief.* New York: Random House.

[33] Carter JP, Saxe GP, Newbold V, Peres CE, Campeau RJ, Bernal- Green L. Hypothesis: dietary management may improve survival from nutritionally linked cancers based on analysis of representative cases. *J Am Coll Nutr* 1993 Jun;12(3):209-26.

[34] Scholz, Mark M.D. Blum, Ralph (2006) "Can Diet Really Control Prostate Cancer?" PCRI Insights, February. vol. 9

meat, poultry, eggs, dairy and sugar.[35]

He immediately went on a macrobiotic diet of whole grains, beans and vegetables. Seven months later, he was well — the aggressive prostate cancer WAS GONE.

Now 64, Dirk is the father of two sons. And he's continued working as an actor and director in TV and film.

As prostate expert Roger Mason put it so aptly in his book *The Natural Prostate Cure,* Dirk is happy and healthy, but *"if he had listened to the doctors, he would have died many years ago as a sexless eunuch in diapers, without testicles."*[36]

Roger Mason is another ardent proponent of the macrobiotic diet for men with ANY kind of prostate problem. As he writes in Chapter Eight of his book, *The Natural Prostate Cure:*

"The most important thing in curing prostate, or any other cancer, is to change your diet and lifestyle and stop eating fats, oils, dairy, poultry, eggs, red meat, sugar and other sweeteners (even honey and maple syrup), tropical foods, hydrogenated oils, preservatives, chemicals, coffee, cigarettes, prescription drugs, and alcohol.

"A diet based on whole grains, beans, most vegetables, some local fruit, and small amounts of seafood (if you are compatible with it), is the way to cure yourself and get well…

"All long-lived people eat a diet based on whole grains, beans, vegetables, local fruits and very little, if any, meat or dairy products. They also eat very low-calorie meals with a fat intake of about 15 percent, generally."[37] [Emphasis added]

You can read more about Roger's specific diet for prostate problems in his book, *The Natural Prostate Cure.*

---

35   Benedict, Dirk (1991) *Confessions of a Kamikaze Cowboy.* Dirk Benedict.

36   Mason, Roger (2000) *The Natural Prostate Cure: A Practical Guide To Using Diet And Supplements.* Roger Mason

37   Mason, Roger (2000) *The Natural Prostate Cure: A Practical Guide To Using Diet And Supplements.* Roger Mason.

The legendary Dr. Dean Ornish watched cancer patients' PSAs decline

Even Dr. Dean Ornish, who's famous for developing the diet that promotes a healthy heart, now believes diet can *ALSO* treat prostate cancer effectively.

In the September, 2005, issue of *The Journal of Urology*, he published the results of his study on diet and lifestyle in 93 prostate cancer patients.[38]

Dr. Ornish gave half of the men a vegetarian, non-dairy diet similar to the macrobiotic diet. He also gave them supplements of antioxidants such as lycopene, selenium and vitamin E. Then he prescribed moderate aerobic exercise and stress management. The other half of the men went untreated.

At the end of one year, the PSAs of the diet-and-lifestyle group had *dropped an average of 4 percent,* or 0.25 ng/ml, while the PSAs of the non-treated group *increased an average of 6 percent,* or 0.38 ng/ml.

Even more telling were Ornish's lab results. He put blood from both groups of men in a Petri dish with prostate cancer cell lines. The blood from the untreated men caused the cancer cells to grow EIGHT TIMES FASTER than did the blood from the diet-and-lifestyle men!

Macrobiotics as a prostate cancer "preventative"

Eating macrobiotically might also help you PREVENT prostate cancer. There's significant research in humans and animals showing that many of the foods in the modern macrobiotic diet are powerful cancer fighters.

For instance, several studies comparing women who eat vegetarian meals with those who

---

38   Ornish, Dean, et al: Intensive lifestyle changes may affect the progression of prostate cancer. *The Journal of Urology* Vol. 174:1065, 2005.

eat traditional western meals show that estrogen metabolism is IMPROVED in the vegetarian group. This reduces the risk of hormone-dependent cancers such as breast and prostate cancer.[39]

Even the American Institute for Cancer Research and the World Cancer Research Fund have reported that eating MORE vegetables and fruit could save MILLIONS of people from getting cancer. In 1997 the two organizations found that simply by improving daily vegetable and fruit consumption from 250g to 400g, an estimated 20 PERCENT *FEWER* PEOPLE would be diagnosed with cancer annually.[40]

Macrobiotics is clearly good cancer prevention. It's also shown to treat both early and advanced prostate cancers. Best of all, it's a diet so you can combine it with other alternative treatments, even with radiation and surgery should you choose. Here's a vital point: You don't need to go to a doctor to take advantage of the healing power of macrobiotic food. There are many books and resources available to help you get started on a macrobiotic diet. If you want more help, you can go to a macrobiotic center or find a macrobiotic counselor to help you craft a macrobiotic diet that suits your specific needs.

For more information:

To find a macrobiotic counselor or center near you, contact:

Kushi Institute
198 Leland Road
Becket, MA 01223
Tel: 1-800-975-8744
Fax: 413-623-8827
Web site: http://www.kushiinstitute.org
E-mail: programs@kushiinstitute.org

The George Ohsawa Macrobiotic Foundation
Web site: http://www.ohsawamacrobiotics.com

Here you can order many macrobiotic books dealing with cancer, including:

Macrobiotic Approach to Cancer — Michio Kushi; 1991; 177 pp.; $13.95. Expanded edition of this health best-seller that aims to prevent and control cancer.

My Beautiful Life: How I Conquered Cancer Naturally — Mina Dobic; 2007; 178 pp.; $15.95. A personal story of insight, courage, and healing from Los Angeles's most expert macrobiotic health consultant.

Recovery from Cancer — Elaine Nussman; 2004; 178 pp.; $14.95.

Basic Macrobiotic Cooking, Revised Edition — Julia Ferré; 2007; 288 pp.; $17.95.

To read excerpts from Dirk Benedict's book, *Confessions of a Kamikaze Cowboy*, or to buy a copy, log onto his Web site: http://www.dirkbenedictcentral.com.

To get Roger Mason's *The Natural Prostate Cure* or *Zen Macrobiotics for Americans,* visit his Web site: www.youngagain.com.

---

39 Goldin BR, et al. Effect of diet on excretion of estrogens in pre- and postmenopausal women. *Cancer Res* 1981 Sep;41(9 Pt 2):3771-3.
Goldin BR, et al. Estrogen excretion patterns and plasma levels in vegetarian and omnivorous women. *N Engl J Med* 1982 Dec 16;307(25):1542-7.
Thomas HV, et al. Endogenous estrogen and postmenopausal breast cancer: a quantitative review. *Cancer Causes Control* 1997 Nov;8(6):922-8.
Key TJ, et al. A prospective study of urinary oestrogen excretion and breast cancer risk. *Br J Cancer* 1996 Jun;73 (12):1615-9.
Adlercreutz H, et al. Determination of urinary lignans and phytoestrogen metabolites, potential antiestrogens and anticarcinogens, in urine of women on various habitual diets. *J Steroid Biochem* 1986 Nov;25(5B):791-7.
Adlercreutz H, et al. Effect of dietary components, including lignans and phytoestrogens, on enterohepatic circulation and liver metabolism of estrogens and on sex hormone binding globulin (SHBG). *J Steroid Biochem* 1987;27(4-6):1135-44.
Ingram D, et al. Case-control study of phyto-oestrogens and breast cancer. *Lancet* 1997 Oct 4;350 (9083):990-4.

40 World Cancer Research Fund [and] American Institute for Cancer Research. Food, nutrition, and the prevention of cancer: a global perspective. Washington (DC): American Institute for Cancer Research; 1997.

Chapter Four

Prostate Cancer Treatment No. 3

The Amazing Non-Toxic Liquid that Killed Virtually 100% of Cancer Cells Within 48 Hours at the National Cancer Institute!

The power of this next alternative cancer treatment is simply astonishing, especially when you consider how simple and safe it is to use on your own, at home.

You see, this treatment doesn't require dramatically changing your diet, or taking several different supplements. This treatment is nothing more than one amazing liquid that's so easy and safe you can give it to a baby, yet it's such a potent cancer killer that the author of one best-selling book on alternative cancer treatments believes it's the *very best* cancer treatment available.

Tanya Harter Pierce, author of *Outsmart Your Cancer*, admitted, "*I could find more complete recoveries from cancer with this treatment called Protocel® than I could find on any other cancer treatment.*"

Even more exciting, a good number of these recoveries are from prostate cancer. And these recoveries aren't just from early prostate cancer either, but advanced cases where aggressive cancer has spread throughout the body. One of the most impressive late-stage recoveries is the story of Herb N.

Herb thought he whipped prostate cancer, but then it came back!

Like many men diagnosed with prostate cancer, Herb[41] underwent a radical prostatectomy (prostate removal surgery). He felt he was in very good hands since the operation was performed by one of the country's foremost prostate doctors at Stanford University Medical Center. After his prostate was removed, Herb was relieved the cancer was gone for good.

Unfortunately, 13 years after the radical operation, Herb's prostate cancer returned. And it came back with a vengeance. His PSA shot up to 135 and he felt pain throughout his body. It's no wonder, his PET scan showed, as he put it, "*widespread bone metastases in my spine, ribs, pelvis and right femur.*"

Herb refused conventional chemotherapy and radiation offered at Stanford. Instead, he decided to seek treatment at an alternative cancer clinic in the U.S. The treatment was natural but expensive (and it wasn't covered by his health insurance). Still, Herb was certain that treating the cancer naturally was the only way he could survive.

Six months later, Herb had a second PET scan. For some reason, the treatment that worked for other types of cancer didn't do a thing against Herb's prostate cancer. The cancer had progressed *even more!* The scan showed "significant increases" in the number of metastases. Herb was disappointed, but not ready to give up. He had recently read Tanya Harter Pierce's book *Outsmart Your Cancer* and decided to try Protocel®.

---

41 Harter Pierce, Tanya, M.A., MFCC (2009) *Outsmart Your Cancer (2nd Edition).* Nevada: Thoughtworks Publishing

Recurrent, metastasized cancer vanishes!

Herb began taking Protocel® at home on his own. Within two weeks, he reported that his pain had diminished and he no longer needed pain killing drugs. He also felt more energetic than he had in months!

After six months on Protocel®, Herb had another PET scan. This time, the results were fantastic. They read *"Marked improvement on the previous pattern of widespread [bone] metastatic disease. No new bone lesions are seen and the previous have nearly resolved."*

Another scan ten months later revealed the news Herb and his family had been waiting for: *There was no evidence of cancer.*

Protocel®: The formula based on a remarkable Nobel Prize winning discovery!

After reviewing reports, it appears to me that Protocel® is entirely unique among alternative cancer treatments. And not just for its simplicity. There are two more important reasons. First of all, Protocel® does not rely on any herbs, vitamins or minerals for anti-cancer activity. Second and most surprising, Protocel® does not rely on boosting the immune system to kill cancer cells.

What does Protocel® do? *Something that's even more effective for many patients who have been failed by other treatments.*

Protocel® is a non-toxic liquid that targets cancer cells biologically, forcing them to shut down, die and disintegrate, according to research published in *Outsmart Your Cancer*. Best of all, the research shows it leaves healthy cells unharmed.

The simplest explanation for Protocel's® cancer-killing success is that cancer cells grow by eating *sugar* while healthy cells eat oxygen. You may recall this idea from earlier, in Chapter Two, when you discovered Dr. Brodie's insulin treatment. Now I want to tell you another important fact about cancer and sugar.

The scientist who discovered what different cells "eat" was Otto Warburg, a German cellular biologist who was born in 1883. The discovery was the breakthrough of his life! In 1931, Warburg won the Nobel Prize! Five years later, another scientist using Warburg's award-winning research into cellular behavior developed Protocel's® unique cancer killing formula.

Jim Sheridan, who was once a researcher at the Detroit Cancer Institute, discovered this amazing formula in his home laboratory. Here's how it works: Protocel® simply blocks cells' ability to feed on sugar. Cancer cells literally starve to death!

American Cancer Society derails safe, cancer-fighting breakthrough

Jim Sheridan was getting amazing results using Protocel® to treat mice with cancer. His studies confirmed Protocel® cured cancer in up to 80 PERCENT of mice without any side effects. Soon, other scientists were interested. Everyone agreed there was enough solid research to begin clinical trials in humans. And that's when the proverbial roof came down.

When the American Cancer Society heard the news, they blocked the clinical program. A few months later, Jim Sheridan was suspiciously fired from the Detroit Institute of Cancer Research and all of his research on Protocel® was reportedly burned!

You have to wonder, why on earth would the American Cancer Society (ACS) do such a thing? Was it pressure by the cancer industry? Fear that Protocel's® success would turn conventional cancer treatment upside down? Probably. Because the only statement the American Cancer Society would make is that they did not approve of the program because *"Jim Sheridan had not proved that he owned the idea."*[42] (Clearly, a ridiculous reason. And if there was such an omission, it could easily be righted with further investigation into Jim Sheridan's research.)

Then, the National Cancer Institute examined Protocel® with astonishing results!

Even though clinical studies never moved forward, all hope was not lost. Studies of Protocel® in cancer cell *lines* would eventually occur years later, at the Natural Cancer Institute (NCI) in 1990. The results were remarkable...

NCI researchers found Protocel® <u>killed virtually 100% of cancer cells within 48 hours.</u> The researchers tested lung cancer cells, melanoma cells, colon cancer cells and ovarian cancer cells. Yet, despite Protocel's® success, the National Cancer Institute has never moved forward with additional research of any kind.

It's important to note that while prostate cancer cells were not among those tested in the National Cancer Institute study, there have been numerous reports of cures from patients with prostate cancer. Those reports also include patients who never had surgery, radiation or chemotherapy for their prostate cancer and are cancer-free to this day! Patients like Albert…

Albert's prostate cancer disappears!

When Albert was 68 years old he was diagnosed with prostate cancer, confirmed by a needle biopsy and five or six prostate tissue samples.[43] Luckily, Albert already knew about Protocel®. He refused surgery, radiation and any other conventional treatment for his cancer. His doctors thought he was nuts to treat his cancer at home, by himself!

Today, five years later, Albert's PSA is stable. He still has his prostate and the cancer is gone. His great results have been proven by his doctor with PSA tests, CT and bone scans, blood work and an MRI.

Alan's prostate cancer is gone, too!

Alan's prostate cancer was also confirmed by a needle biopsy.[44] However, the biopsy caused a serious infection that made Alan severely ill. It took him weeks to recover and reinforced his inclination to avoid conventional treatments. Instead he took Protocel® at home to fight his prostate tumor.

One year after he started taking Protocel, tests revealed he was cancer-free. His PSA has dropped from 11.1 to 2.5 and all diagnostic tests indicate "no clinical signs" of cancer.

How to take Protocel® for prostate cancer

Protocel appears effective in both advanced and early prostate cancers. As with most alternative therapies, the earlier you begin treatment the higher your chances of success.

There are two different Protocel® formulas, Protocel® Formula 50 and Protocel® Formula 23. Each formula works better for certain kinds of cancer. For prostate cancer, Protocel® Formula 23 is recommended. It is readily available today and costs about $110 a bottle for a month and a half's supply.

Protocel® Formula 23 is very easy to take, and very little is required. Regular dosing instructions are generally between ¼ and ½ a teaspoon. This dose is taken five times a day with each dose spaced out over a 24 hour period.

The idea, says Tanya Harter Pierce, is never to go more than six hours between any two doses so you block cancer cells from getting any

---

[42] Harter Pierce, Tanya, M.A., MFCC (2009) *Outsmart Your Cancer (2nd Edition)*. Nevada: Thoughtworks Publishing

[43] Harter Pierce, Tanya, M.A., MFCC (2009) *Outsmart Your Cancer (2nd Edition)*. Nevada: Thoughtworks Publishing.

[44] Harter Pierce, Tanya, M.A., MFCC (2009) *Outsmart Your Cancer (2nd Edition)*. Nevada: Thoughtworks Publishing.

nourishment. For example, you could take the formula at 7 a.m., 11:30 a.m., 4 p.m., 8:30 p.m., and 2 a.m. (yes, you have to set an alarm and wake up for that middle of the night dose!)

Important: Protocel® is not compatible with other natural treatments

As you can see, taking Protocel® is relatively simple. However, the formula's biological effects on cancer cells are quite complex. Therefore, Protocel® should not be taken with any other natural treatments, not even ordinary vitamins and minerals in a multi-vitamin!

In her book, *Outsmart Your Cancer*, Tanya Harter Pierce provides a long list of therapies to avoid while using Protocel®. Among the most common: Vitamin C, Vitamin E, Selenium, Fish Oil, CoQ10, and Ginseng. Essentially, you don't want to take anything "extra" while you're taking Protocel®.

It's also important, says Tanya, to drink plenty of water (at least a half gallon a day) and stay regular, using laxatives if necessary. Both will help your body process and eliminate dead cancer cells.

Editorial note: After reading the available research on Protocel® and hearing from men who have taken Protocel® for prostate cancer and other cancers, I've come to the conclusion that Protocel® works very well for certain men and not very well for others.

From what I've learned, if Protocel® is going to work to cure your prostate cancer then it will work relatively quickly — within a matter of months. You can get regular diagnostic testing after starting Protocel® or any other treatment to monitor your progress. Also, I discovered that many men with prostate cancer have reported an increase in their PSA after they begin taking Protocel®. This is believed to be a "healing crisis" and results from cancer cells quickly dying off.

Something else to consider: While many patients who report success with Protocel® do not change their diets substantially, if I was battling prostate cancer I would increase my intake of vegetables and fruit and decrease my intake of meat and dairy products to help my body fight the disease.

For more information:

Tanya Harter Pierce's book, *Outsmart Your Cancer*, is considered the definitive guide to using Protocel® to treat cancer. It is recommended by Jim Sheridan's family and licensed Protocel® distributors. I strongly encourage picking up a copy should you choose to take Protocel® for your prostate cancer. You can purchase a copy for $26.95 from our website: http://www.cancerdefeated.com/OYC/.

Protocel® is sold through licensed distributors in the United States and internationally. For U.S. purchases contact:

Vitamin Depot
Tel: 330-634-0008
Web: www.yourvitamindepot.com
For questions ask for Dr. Kimberly Cassidy (Doctor of Naturopathy)

Renewal and Wellness, LLC
Tel: 888-581-4442
Web: http://www.webnd.com

For international purchases contact:

Go-Global Health Marketing, Inc.
Customer Service
email: sales@Protocelglobal.com
Web: www.Protocelglobal.com

Chapter Five

Prostate Cancer Treatment No. 4

Flood Your Body with Oxygen and Cancer Cells Will Die On Contact: The Budwig Protocol

When "Bill" (not his real name) was diagnosed with prostate cancer, he learned it had spread outside his prostate and into his *spine*. Sadly, Bill's doctors told him his disease was so advanced that he should get his affairs in order and prepare for the end. But Bill's wife refused to give up hope and began investigating alternative treatments.

She learned about a simple nutritional protocol developed by a German biochemist that has worked wonders for probably thousands of prostate cancer patients. And she persuaded Bill to try it. Lo and behold, he started feeling better *every day*.

In six months, Bill's "hopeless" prostate cancer was gone!

Bill went back to his doctor's office six months later. The doctor couldn't believe he was still alive, much less looking so good! The doctor immediately examined Bill's prostate and put him through all the ordinary diagnostic tests for cancer. EVERY SINGLE TEST CAME BACK NEGATIVE! That's right, the advanced prostate cancer that had spread throughout Bill's body had simply vanished.

Bill is *still* cancer-free, three years and counting. He's such a believer in this nutritional protocol that he uses it *every day* to make sure the cancer doesn't come back. Thank goodness this protocol is easy to stick with. It doesn't require overhauling your diet — you just add two "foods" you can get at any natural health food store.

The incredible cancer-killing power of flaxseed oil and cottage cheese

That's right, flaxseed oil and cottage cheese! That combination might not get your taste buds' attention, but it certainly gets the attention of cancer cells. This unique combination of foods has the *natural power* to KILL THEM!

German biochemist Dr. Johanna Budwig[45] was the first to discover this, after noticing that people with chronic illnesses such as cancer and arthritis have very *low* levels of omega-3 fatty acids in their blood.

Around 1951, she found a simple way to reintroduce these fats into the bloodstream. She discovered that the human body *easily* absorbs the omega-3 fats and protein naturally present in flaxseed oil and cottage cheese. What happened next was amazing:

Cancer cells fell apart and died!

Dr. Budwig noticed that the omega-3 fats and protein from flaxseed oil and cottage cheese easily reached cancer cells, flooding them with oxygen, which attacks them. The result? Cancer cells simply <u>fell apart and died.</u> It's a process

---

45 "The Story and Studies of Johanna Budwig," www.budwig-flax.com

called *"oxidation."*

Modern medicine has known about the power of oxidation since the 1930's. That's when science first discovered that oxidation can make *normal cells healthier* and *wipe out cancer cells*.

But Dr. Budwig is one of only a few doctors who've actually taken advantage of this simple process to cure cancer! And her brilliant discoveries haven't gone unnoticed: She's been nominated for the Nobel Prize *seven times*.

Of course, conventional medicine still laughs off her simple cancer cure as sheer quackery. But patients who've tried it are happily getting the last laugh! Many of them have gotten incredible results in just *days* or *weeks* when NOTHING ELSE worked to stop their cancers — especially prostate cancer.

David's advanced prostate cancer disappears!

In my research I uncovered several reports from a German naturopath who has set up a Web Site to inform others on the Budwig Protocol.[46] That's where I learned about "Bill" and also "David" (not his real name). David was stricken with advanced prostate cancer. He was in terrible pain, a common symptom for men in the late stages of the disease. Even worse, his doctors could no longer help him. All he could do was lie on the couch and *suffer*. His daughter could hardly stand it.

She'd heard about the flaxseed oil and started giving it to him. In a few weeks, this once-dying man was out driving his truck again. He was feeling worlds better. He was even calling his friends to report his amazing recovery with this strange natural treatment.

Frank's PSA drops 60 points in 90 days!

From this naturopath I also discovered "Frank" (not his real name), who was 75 when he learned his PSA was almost as high as his age — a horrific 73. He decided to try the flaxseed-oil-and-cottage-cheese cure.

For the next three months he used it every day, while also eating mostly raw fruits and vegetables. At the end of three months, Frank's PSA had dropped to an unbelievable 13 — *a 60-point drop in just 90 days!*

There are many more stories of prostate cancer recoveries like Bill's, David's and Frank's. One of the most famous is Cliff Beckwith's. According to a web site Cliff began, he lived an active life *with advanced prostate cancer* for an incredible 17 years after doctors said he'd die.

Cliff always maintained that the Budwig Protocol saved his life. He was such an advocate that he started making audio tapes, and eventually launched his web site to help other men discover the flaxseed-oil-and-cottage-cheese treatment.

Sadly, Cliff passed away in April, 2007, nearly two decades after his "hopeless" diagnosis. His family has kept his web site intact to help other men struggling with prostate cancer. You can find it at http://www.beckwithfamily.com. There, you'll discover other testimonials from men who had prostate cancer and used the Budwig Protocol to send it into remission.

Besides numerous prostate cancer patients, many renowned cancer experts also believe in the curative powers of the Budwig Protocol.

Natural health M.D. praises the Budwig Protocol for cancer!

In a 1990 issue of the *Townsend Letter for Doctors & Patients*, Dr. Dan C. Roehm, M.D., F.A.C.P., an oncologist and former cardiologist,

---
46 "Budwig Protocol." www.healingcancernaturally.com

raved about the "immediate" curative effects of the Budwig Protocol:

"This diet is far and away the most successful anti-cancer diet in the world. What she [Dr. Johanna Budwig] has demonstrated to my initial disbelief, but lately to my complete satisfaction in my practice, is: CANCER IS EASILY CURABLE.

"*The treatment is dietary/lifestyle, the response is immediate; the cancer cell is weak and vulnerable; the precise biochemical breakdown point was identified by her in 1951 and is specifically correctable, in vitro (test tube) as well as in vivo (real). I only wish that all my patients had a PhD in Biochemistry and Quantum Physics to enable them to see how with such consummate skill this diet was put together. It is a wonder.*"[47] [Emphasis added]

Another leading advocate of the Budwig Protocol is cancer author and radio commentator Bill Henderson.

Bill has written repeatedly about how he himself takes flaxseed oil and cottage cheese every single day to prevent prostate cancer (or any other cancer) from growing in his body.

In his book *Cancer-Free*, Bill points out that when people use it correctly, the Budwig Protocol has shown a SUCCESS RATE OF 90 PERCENT in clinical research. And this research included patients who'd tried radiation and surgery, and their doctors couldn't help them.[48]

How to use the Budwig Protocol the *right* way

One thing that's clear in all the articles and books I've read on the Budwig Protocol is that you must use the EXACT ingredients in the EXACT WAY that Dr. Budwig recommends in order for the treatment to work.

Her protocol calls for using quark (a dairy food readily available in Europe, but less so in the USA), cottage cheese or yogurt. Most Americans use cottage cheese. Choose an organic, preservative-free brand with one or two percent fat. Mix two-thirds of a cup with six tablespoons of high-quality flaxseed oil (stored in your refrigerator). This is your daily dose.

If you choose yogurt, Dr. Budwig recommends *tripling* the amount. In other words, you've got to eat *two* cups of yogurt with six tablespoons of flaxseed oil.

Though some patients say the cottage cheese/oil mixture is an acquired taste, others enjoy it. Many have their cottage cheese and flaxseed oil for breakfast.

For example, Bill Henderson makes a fruit smoothie with it every day. If you choose to make a smoothie like he does, make sure you add the flaxseed oil, *blending it only by hand,* AFTER you've mixed all the other ingredients in your blender. In other words, NEVER blend the oil in the blender! Here's why:

Dr. Budwig and others report that ANY type of heat (even from the blender motor) can destroy the flaxseed oil's omega-3 content and render it useless. This is one reason why it's imperative that you buy a fresh, high-quality oil (experts often recommend Barleans brand) and store it properly in your refrigerator.

Editorial note: The Budwig Protocol does not require changing your diet, other than adding the necessary flaxseed oil and cottage cheese combination. However, if it were me I would adopt elements of proven cancer fighting diets which include high amounts of fresh vegetables and fruits and less meat and dairy products.

---

[47] Henderson, Bill (2008) *Cancer-Free (Third Edition)* Booklocker, Inc.

[48] Henderson, Bill (2008) *Cancer-Free (Third Edition)* Booklocker, Inc.

For more information:

Flax Oil As a True Aid Against Arthritis, Heart Infarction, Cancer and Other Diseases by Dr. Johanna Budwig (available on Amazon)

The Oil-Protein Diet Cookbook by Dr. Johanna Budwig (available on Amazon)

The Budwig Cancer & Coronary Heart Disease Prevention Diet: The Revolutionary Diet from Dr. Johanna Budwig, the Woman Who Discovered Omega-3s by Dr. Johanna Budwig (available on Amazon)

Online chat group for the Budwig Protocol: FlaxSeedOil2@yahoogroups.com

High-quality flaxseed oil is available from Barleans: http://www.barleans.com/

Cliff Beckwith Web site: http://www.beckwithfamily.com

Chapter Six

Prostate Cancer Treatment No. 5

Cutting-Edge Sound Treatment Melts Away Early Prostate Cancer! High-Intensity Focused Ultrasound — HIFU

Many men, when they hear the dreaded "C-word," just want to get the cancer cut out as soon as possible — no matter what. And, of course, plenty of conventional doctors are willing to tell them that it's a good idea. That can be a mistake, in my view.

Surgery ISN'T necessarily your best option (see Chapter Nine), but if you decide it is, I've got a much gentler, kinder "surgery" for you. In fact, some patients don't consider this breakthrough surgery at all, but a simple scalpel-less procedure that gets rid of the cancer without getting rid of the prostate!

This breakthrough is a new treatment for prostate cancer called *High-Intensity Focused Ultrasound* or HIFU (pronounced HIGH-foo).

Instead of a scalpel, this treatment uses acoustic *sound waves* to generate thermal (heat) energy that melts away prostate cancer. Yes, I said *melts*: The acoustic sound waves super-heat the prostate to a whopping 194 degrees Fahrenheit, killing prostate cancer cells.

How <u>sound</u> kills cancer cells

This treatment is based on the same principle as hyperthermia (heat) treatments. Cancer clinics throughout Germany use those treatments to treat all sorts of cancers. The principle is that *heat kills cancer cells.*

German doctors using hyperthermia heat regions of the patient's body where cancer exists to temperatures upwards of 109 degrees Fahrenheit. But HIFU is much more specific. It heats ONLY the prostate with pinpoint accuracy, so doctors can safely use much, much higher temperatures, giving cancer an even slimmer chance of surviving.

Researchers have found that HIFU kills prostate cancer WITHOUT causing the common side effects that conventional surgery and radiation cause, such as impotence and urinary incontinence. The reason is that, unlike prostate surgery and radiation, the nerves necessary for erection and bladder control are not affected by HIFU in any way. More on this in a minute, but first I want to tell you what men experience during HIFU.

The entire HIFU treatment is scalpel-less. It takes about two to three-and-a-half hours, and is done on an outpatient basis. You will undergo general anesthesia during the procedure and you'll need a catheter for a week or so after treatment. However, most patients usually resume their normal, active lives within two days, and sometimes sooner. Just ask Gary Crissman.

HIFU is a pain-free "breeze"

Gary Crissman was 54 when he was diagnosed with prostate cancer. Worried that prostate surgery would leave him impotent and in diapers for the rest of his life, he opted for HIFU.

"I didn't want to have the problem of potentially leaking, and I didn't want to have the problem of erectile dysfunction," Gary told a *New York Times* reporter in 2008.[49] Calling the painless procedure a "breeze," Gary recounted how he "celebrated" getting rid of his prostate cancer that very SAME NIGHT with a buffet dinner at his hotel.

"Procedure is very easy" says Greg

Another patient named Greg said having HIFU was much, much easier than any kind of prostate surgery. He posted a report of his experience on an online blog:

"The procedure is very easy. You can arrive the day before the procedure and travel home the next day if you want. Just four hours after the procedure, we walked to the marina for dinner. The day after the procedure, my wife and I did a walking tour of [the city], and we probably walked three miles. Other than a catheter, you don't feel any different after the procedure than before, other than relieved… All my functions are normal…I have no urinary function issues at all. I have no impotency issues, either."[50]

Sound breakthrough discovered at Indiana University

HIFU is a relatively new procedure, but the breakthrough behind it is more than 50 years old. Research began at Indiana University in Bloomington in the 1950's. They studied a special ultrasound device to see if it could deliver enough thermal energy to destroy cancer. Results showed that <u>it could in fact kill cancer cells</u>. And the sound treatment was *safe* and doctors could *repeat* it if cancer recurred.

In 1995, a study on modern-day HIFU at the university revealed something even more spectacular: Researchers discovered they could treat the WHOLE PROSTATE *without* damaging the prostate capsule (the membrane that surrounds the prostate).[51]

This is a tremendous advantage over traditional prostate surgeries that damage the prostate membrane. When the membrane is damaged, often the nerves necessary for erection and the urinary sphincter necessary for bladder control are damaged too. That's why so many men are becoming impotent and incontinent after conventional prostate treatments!

Not only that, urologists say damaging the prostate membrane can "spill" cancer cells into the patient's bloodstream and spread the disease!

"The ability to treat the prostate with virtually no disruption of the capsule avoids unnecessary spillage of cancer cells that is common to radical prostatectomy," says Dr. Ronald Wheeler, a urologist and HIFU practitioner at the Diagnostic Center for Disease in Sarasota, Florida.[52]

The 1995 study also found another wonderful benefit. HIFU *doesn't* damage the patient's rectal wall. Damaging it can cause fecal incontinence. This is a tragic and little-known side effect of conventional IMRT and brachytherapy, with or without External Beam or Proton Beam. These amazing benefits of the HIFU approach bear repeating…

Men Keep Their Sexual Function, Bladder and Bowel Control

At first it was hard for me to understand how HIFU could destroy cancerous prostate cells and tissue without at least diminishing sexual function. But then I heard Dr. Wheeler's explanation (and learned a lot more about male

---

49 Saul, Stephanie "Despite Doubts, Cancer Therapy Draws Patients." *The New York Times* January 18, 2008

50 Greg, Personal Blog Post. http://www.cancercompass.com/messages/Greg1961, Dec 29, 2007

51 HIFU Care Center. www.hifucarecenter.com

52 Wheeler, Ronald M.D. (1998-2010) "Sexual Potency Is Maintained by Design As the Neurovascular Bundles Are Mapped out of the Treatment Plan." Florida: Diagnostic Center for Disease.

anatomy) and it all made sense.

The tissues SURROUNDING your prostate are what's important to erectile function and bladder control — not the prostate itself. Right outside the prostate membrane are nerves necessary to achieve erection. This is also where the urinary sphincter for bladder control is located.

According to Dr. Wheeler, surgery and radiation can damage these areas but the HIFU procedure is far more precise than any kind of radiation or surgical treatment — even more precise than those brand new robotic surgeries, guided by the Da Vinci Robot.® [53] HIFU never reaches outside the prostate membrane so these nerves and the urinary sphincter remain untouched.[54]

Men have the exact same sexual and bladder function *after* HIFU as they had *before*. The only difference is that you may have less ejaculatory fluid. This is due to cell death within the prostate. Regardless, you'll likely maintain your fertility. Dr. Wheeler's office reports that his patients' ejaculatory fluids *still* contain live sperm. Tests they've done on the fluid of post-HIFU men in their 70's have proven it.

Clinical study results: HIFU safe and effective

Independent clinical studies performed in Germany and Japan reveal that HIFU *is a safe and effective* treatment for prostate cancer.

In Germany, 146 men with Gleason scores of 7 or lower and PSAs of 15 ng/ml or lower were treated with HIFU. Two years later, 93.4 PERCENT HAD NEGATIVE BIOPSIES and 87 percent had PSA levels under 1.0![55] [A Gleason score is used to evaluate the aggressiveness of prostate cancer.]

Japanese researchers performed their own study and concluded that *"High-intensity focused ultrasound therapy appears to be a safe and efficacious minimally invasive therapy for patients with localized prostate cancer."*[56]

"Localized" prostate cancer means prostate cancer that hasn't spread. Japanese researchers found that men with PSA levels under 10 *before* the procedure had a 94 PERCENT chance of surviving at least three years after treatment.

HIFU: A wonderful new option for early prostate cancer

There are many success stories of men who appear to have cured their prostate cancers completely, with no debilitating side effects, using HIFU. The best results are in men with *early-stage* prostate cancer. Unfortunately, men who have more advanced cases aren't faring as well.

The same research in Germany and Japan shows that when the cancer has spread *outside* the man's prostate, or he has a higher PSA or Gleason score, HIFU treatment isn't as successful. *Why?*

Dr. Wheeler reports that as prostate cancer advances, calcified stones form in your prostate. These stones can *"prevent the focused energy from getting to tissue on the other side"* or worse, the sound energy can be reflected back toward the

---

53   Wheeler, Ronald M.D. (1998-2010) "Sexual Potency Is Maintained by Design As the Neurovascular Bundles Are Mapped out of the Treatment Plan." Florida: Diagnostic Center for Disease.

54   Wheeler, Ronald M.D. (1998-2010) "Sexual Potency Is Maintained by Design As the Neurovascular Bundles Are Mapped out of the Treatment Plan." Florida: Diagnostic Center for Disease.

---

55   Blana A, Walter B, Rogenhofer S, Wieland WF. Department of Urology, University of Regensburg, St. Josef Hospital, Regensburg, Germany. High-intensity focused ultrasound for the treatment of localized prostate cancer: 5-year experience. *Urology*. 2004 Feb;63(2):297-300.

56   Uchida T, Shoji S, Nakano M, Hongo S, Nitta M, Murota A, Nagata Y. *Department of Urology*, Tokai University Hachioji Hospital, Hachioji, Tokyo, Japan. Transrectal high-intensity focused ultrasound for the treatment of localized prostate cancer: eight-year experience. *Int J Urol*. 2009 Nov;16(11):881-6.

rectal wall.[57] In other words, the sound energy is diffused and parts of the prostate never reach the temperature necessary for cancer cells to die.

The other interesting part of the story is what happens when you DO send HIFU's energy outside the prostate. Remember, that's where nerves for erectile function and bladder control are located. It seems that in some men with more advanced cancers, HIFU is resulting in the SAME side effects as traditional prostate therapies such as incontinence and sexual dysfunction!

We might conclude that when HIFU is used to treat cancer that lies OUTSIDE the prostate capsule, as it often does in advanced cases, HIFU's heat destroys healthy tissues right along with cancerous ones. From the research it's clear to me that HIFU may not be for everyone.

"We must not use the one-size-fits-all mentality with HIFU, as often times occurs with radical prostatectomy," Dr. Wheeler cautions. *"As skilled surgeons, we must be able to accept that all men with prostate cancer will not be viable candidates for HIFU for a variety of reasons, and therefore, must encourage them to treat their disease with an alternative."*[58]

Who should get HIFU — and who shouldn't

Dr. Thomas Gardner, M.D., agrees with Dr. Wheeler. Dr. Gardner is a professor of urology and one of the researchers at Indiana University School Medicine who was involved in FDA clinical trials of HIFU.

In an interview in Bottom Line's *Daily Health* newsletter, Dr. Gardner says HIFU can be an amazing treatment *"in the right hands, among appropriate patients."*[59] He recommends HIFU *only* for men who have:

- early-stage (T1 or T2) prostate cancer
- localized tumors that haven't spread outside the prostate
- a Gleason score of six or lower
- a PSA level under 10 ng/ml
- a prostate that's no larger than 40cc in volume

Is HIFU a long-term cure for early prostate cancer?

HIFU is still a very new treatment and much of the research in prostate cancer patients is little more than 10 years old, so no long-term cure rates are available.

Some experts caution that HIFU may not *completely* cure prostate cancer, because there've been some cases of recurrence. Dr. Wheeler believes the explanation is simple: *Prostate cancer recurs when HIFU isn't used on "carefully selected" patients.*[60] His office reports that when men are properly qualified the cancer DOES NOT RETURN.

Other experts point to the simplicity of the treatment and how you can receive it again and again to safely melt away recurring prostate cancers. In fact, research suggests that some men might *need* more than one treatment to get rid of their prostate cancer completely.

Current FDA clinical trials

HIFU is currently undergoing two different FDA-approved clinical trials in the USA. The first trial is of *primary organ-confined* or localized prostate cancer in 466 men being treated at 24 different treatment centers. A second trial will

---

57 Wheeler, Ronald M.D. (1998-2010) "Why HIFU Fails to Cure Prostate Cancer. Florida: Diagnostic Center for Disease." Reprinted with permission.

58 Wheeler, Ronald M.D. (1998-2010) "Sexual Potency Is Maintained by Design As the Neurovascular Bundles Are Mapped out of the Treatment Plan." Florida: Diagnostic Center for Disease. Reprinted with permission.

59 "Ultrasound Treatment for Prostate Cancer." *Bottom Line's: Daily Health News.* Tuesday, May 6, 2008.

60 Wheeler, Ronald M.D. (1998-2010) "Why HIFU Fails to Cure Prostate Cancer. Florida: Diagnostic Center for Disease." Reprinted with permission.

look at men suffering *recurrent* prostate cancer who've already tried conventional external-beam radiation therapy that didn't help them.

Though no results of these trials have been released, the medical monitor of the trials, Dr. Herbert Lepor, Chairman of Urology at NYU School of Medicine, has been quoted as saying, *"I have personally reviewed the preliminary data and observed the Sonablate® 500 [HIFU] in action and I am impressed with this advanced technology."*[61]

How to get HIFU

Currently, the U.S. Government approves HIFU only for "investigational" use. So to get it in the USA you must enroll in a clinical trial, such as those being performed by the FDA.

Fortunately, U.S. HIFU, the company that owns the Sonablate® 500 HIFU technology, has 100 treatment centers worldwide, including centers in Mexico, Canada, Costa Rica, South Africa and the Caribbean.

Gary and Greg, whom I mentioned earlier, both visited the center in Puerto Vallarta, Mexico, where Board Certified Urologist Dr. Stephen Scionti regularly travels from his practice in South Carolina to perform the procedure.

Other Americans such as Richard Brightmire have traveled to the Cancun, Mexico center. He told his story on ABC's "Nightline" in June, 2008. According to the broadcast, four months after *his* HIFU treatment, his PSA had plummeted to *zero* and his quality of life was perfectly "normal."

"I'm doing fine since the HIFU procedure. Everything is back to normal," Brightmire said. *"For me, I went with the procedure because of the results outside the U.S. that show it to be non-invasive and show a lower risk of long-term hospitalization, and a lower risk of incontinence as well as impotence, especially compared to surgery and other treatments available today."*[62]

With a price tag of $25,000-$30,000, HIFU treatment certainly isn't cheap. And because it's not approved by the FDA, your insurance company won't automatically cover the cost.

But according to the U.S. HIFU's Web site, *"Several patients have been able to receive full reimbursement from their insurance company. People have been successful by filing a claim through an independent claims filing service. Patients are given a detailed receipt after the procedure to assist in filing and for tax purposes… You may be able to deduct HIFU as a medical expense on your taxes…"*[63]

For more information:

Watch a 3-D animation of the HIFU procedure here:

http://www.panamhifu.com

Stephen M. Scionti, M.D.
Minimally Invasive Prostate Cancer Specialist
Coastal Carolina Urology Group, LLC
8 Hospital Center Boulevard, Suite 150
Hilton Head Island, SC 29926
Toll-free: 866-422-2284
Fax: 843-342-7640
Web site: www.HIFUcarecenter.com
Web site: www.cryocarecenter.com

Ronald Wheeler, M.D.
Urologist and Director of the Diagnostic Center for Disease
1250 South Tamiami Trail, Suite 101 N
Sarasota, FL 34239
Tel: 941-957-0007
Toll-free: 877-766-8400
Fax: 941-957-1033
E-mail: staff@mrisusa.com
Web site: http://www.ronaldwheeler.com

---

61 United States HIFU, www.ushifu.com
62 United States HIFU, www.ushifu.com
63 United States HIFU, www.ushifu.com

To read more of what Dr. Wheeler says about HIFU, see his article "Sexual Potency is Maintained by Design as the Neurovascular Bundles are Mapped Out of the Treatment Plan" online at http://www.panamhifu.com/why_hifu_fails.asp#FDA_approval

U. S. HIFU
Web site: www.ushifu.com

If patients meet the enrollment criteria, they might qualify to enroll in the U.S. HIFU clinical trials. For more information about the clinical trials' eligibility criteria, call toll-free 1-888-874-4384.

Chapter Seven

Early Detection of Prostate Cancer

The Problem with PSAs and the Test That's Working Better

Doctors have recommended the Prostate-Specific Antigen (PSA) test for all men 40 and older since 1988. When the test was first introduced, doctors were thrilled. They had high hopes that early detection of prostate cancer would save more lives.

But it's become clear that the PSA test has a MAJOR drawback: *Too many false positives — i.e., erroneous test results that say patients have cancer.* And men are being put through needless, painful biopsies — sometimes six or more — plus much emotional trauma, when they don't even *have* prostate cancer!

Up to 70 percent of men *without* prostate cancer are getting *positive* PSA test results!

Research proves that having a high or positive PSA test result by no means proves you have cancer. Many other non-cancerous prostate conditions can raise your prostate-specific antigen. For example, an enlarged prostate (BPH) or inflammation and infection of the prostate (prostatitis) can send your PSA through the roof.

In his book *Cancer-Free*, Bill Henderson reports that up to 70 PERCENT OF MEN with elevated PSA levels turn out NOT to have prostate cancer (i.e., false positives.) Bill himself has reported that he's had high PSA levels, but he doesn't have prostate cancer.[64]

Researchers at the Dana-Farber Cancer Institute at Harvard Medical School recently studied the problem. In a review of years of research, they documented that 50 percent of ALL MEN with high PSAs don't have prostate cancer.[65]

So what *do* these men have? Usually, *prostatitis*.

Prostatitis: Often misdiagnosed as prostate cancer

Urologist Dr. Ronald Wheeler has written extensively on the problem of men with high PSAs being treated for prostate cancer, when in fact they might have a prostate infection or prostatitis. In his article, "PSA: A Barometer to Prostate Health or a License to Biopsy," he writes:

"For the most part, we lack the ability to judge which patients [with high PSAs] are truly at risk [for prostate cancer] and which ones are not. My belief is that there is a means to differentiate patients at risk with an elevated PSA from the group that has little or no risk. Recognition that PSA is driven primarily by prostatitis [inflammation/infection] will allow for

---

[64] Henderson, Bill (2008) *Cancer-Free (Third Edition)* Booklocker, Inc.

[65] Garnick MB. The dilemmas of prostate cancer. Dana Farber Cancer Institute, Harvard Medical School *Sci Am.* 1994 Apr;270(4):72-81. Review. No abstract available.

a more conservative approach [in prostate cancer treatment]."[66] [Emphasis added]

If you discover you have a high PSA, the first thing to rule out is prostatitis, Dr. Wheeler advises. Your doctor does this with a simple manual test called an *"expressed prostatic secretion"* or EPS. It's commonly known as "milking" the prostate. Your doctor will test your prostate secretion for bacterial infection. If it turns out you DO have prostatitis, you'll certainly breathe a sigh of relief that it's not cancer.

But, adds Dr. Wheeler, you shouldn't take prostatitis lightly. It's a warning sign of possible FUTURE cancer. He writes:

"Prostatitis is also an epidemic disease and associated with virtually all cases of prostate cancer. To state further, we must recognize that antibiotics have limitations and work minimally to ameliorate chronic prostatitis as noted in Campbell's Urology, the reference text... Physicians must also be willing to decrease the number of prescriptions written for antibiotics, thereby providing impetus for the use of non-traditional, complementary alternative treatment methodologies."[67]

Treating prostatitis naturally

Dr. Wheeler believes doctors can treat most cases of prostatitis without antibiotics, using natural nutritional therapies. He recommends that patients with prostatitis take a blend of nutritional anti-inflammatories, immune-boosters, herbs, vitamins, minerals and antioxidants. The nutrients include:

- vitamin C
- vitamin E
- vitamin B6
- zinc
- selenium
- saw palmetto
- pygeum
- pumpkin seeds
- stinging nettle

Dr. Wheeler has reported such success with this nutritional approach that he's patented a formula with these nutrients called Peenuts®. Several clinical studies have shown wonderful results in men with prostatitis and BPH.

Patented Peenuts® improves urinary symptoms

In one randomized, double-blind, placebo-controlled study, Peenuts® *"improved ability to decrease the signs and symptoms associated with an enlarged prostate or prostatitis."*[68]

More specifically, ALL the men in the Peenuts® study experienced improved urinary symptoms, such as less frequency, less pain and less dribbling. A whopping 69 percent of them improved in either six or seven of the seven categories measured — in other words, most men's symptoms improved across the board! By the way, these "categories" are based on the IPSS-Index or AUA Symptom Index that doctors use to diagnose prostate problems.

But it's not just one study. In a clinical follow-up to the study, more than 300 men got similar results. The average improvement in their urinary-symptoms scores was a dramatic 11 points. But that's not all…

---

66   Wheeler, Ronald M.D. (1998-2010) "PSA — A Barometer of Prostate Health Or a License to Biopsy." Florida: Diagnostic Center for Disease. Reprinted with permission.

67   Wheeler, Ronald M.D. (1998-2010) "PSA — A Barometer of Prostate Health Or a License to Biopsy." Florida: Diagnostic Center for Disease. Reprinted with permission.

68   Peenuts®, http://www.peenuts.com/peenuts.asp

Patented Peenuts® reduces inflammation

The PSAs of ALL patients studied improved an average of *49 PERCENT!* Meanwhile, the EPS, the most sensitive "marker" for prostatitis, showed a 66 percent drop in white blood cells — a GOOD thing, because it means a drop in inflammation. Best of all, there were *"no side effects or drug interactions noted during testing or clinical follow-up."*[69]

If you want to learn more about Peenuts® or the ingredients in the formula, visit the Web site: www.peenuts.com.

Here's something else that's important to note: In his articles, Dr. Wheeler calls the PSA *"the barometer of prostate health"* and NOT a diagnostic test for prostate cancer. The research shows he's onto something. Urgent new studies reveal that when it comes to prostate cancer, the PSA test has made *little or no difference* in saving men's lives.

Brand-new studies reveal PSA testing *not* saving lives!

Two large, long-term, multi-center studies just published in the *New England Journal of Medicine* show the PSA test provides LITTLE IF ANY reduction in the number of deaths from prostate cancer. That's right, the PSA test has made almost NO DIFFERENCE at all in saving men's lives! And these studies were *massive*.

The first study involved 182,000 men in seven European countries.[70] The second was done by the National Cancer Institute on 77,000 men in the USA.

In the studies, scientists randomly assigned men to receive either (1) no screening or (2) screening with the PSA. Then they monitored the men for 10 years. After seven years, the U.S. researchers made a shocking discovery: The *unscreened group* had a death rate 13 PERCENT LOWER than the screened group!

Almost three years later, after they'd followed most of the men for 10 years, the U.S. researchers concluded there was no *real* reduction in deaths from prostate cancer with PSA screening.

In Europe, the men in the study fared little better.

PSA tests saved only seven lives for every 10,000 men screened!

The PSA-screened groups had a 20 PERCENT REDUCTION in death rate. This sounds somewhat significant, but when you look at the actual numbers, only *seven* men's lives were saved for every 10,000 men screened!

Dr. Otis Brawley, the chief medical officer of the American Cancer Society, told the *New York Times* the studies were *"some of the most important studies in the history of men's health"!*

And then he drove the final nail into the PSA's coffin, exclaiming that benefits of screening are *"modest at best and with a greater downside than any other cancer we screen for."*[71] And this from a mainstream doctor!

But there's *another* problem with the PSA test that conventional doctors aren't talking about at all.

PSA test *MISSES* 15 percent or more of prostate cancers!

Ironically, although the PSA appears to be *overly sensitive* in some cases, in others it's *not sensitive enough* to detect prostate cancer!

In his book *Cancer-Free*, Bill Henderson

---

69 Peenuts®, http://www.peenuts.com/peenuts.asp

70 Schröder FH, et al. Department of Urology, Erasmus Medical Center, Rotterdam, The Netherlands. Screening and prostate-cancer mortality in a randomized European study. N Engl J Med. 2009 Mar 26;360(13):1320-8. Epub 2009 Mar 18.

71 Kolata, Gina (2009) "Review of prostate cancer screening, Prostate Test Found to Save Few Lives." The New York Times

reveals an interesting study he came across in Dr. Robert Rowen's *Second Opinion* newsletter:

"Researchers followed 9,459 men who had annual PSA tests. Of this group, 2,950 had test results showing very healthy prostates," said Dr. Rowen. *"But when these 'healthy' men underwent biopsies, a whopping 15 percent tested positive for cancer! Many had high-grade cancer. And the PSA test missed it in all of them!*

"And the incidence of false negatives may be even higher. You see, prostate biopsies are taken by random needle jabs into the gland. No matter how many sticks are made, there's no way to know if cancer lurks outside the needle track. Bottom line: Don't rely on PSA to tell you whether or not you have cancer. Focus instead on other diagnostic tests."[72]

I agree with Dr. Rowen and Bill Henderson. If your PSA is higher than normal and you've ruled out prostatitis, you might want to consider *other* diagnostic tests for prostate cancer. In fact, there's one VERY IMPORTANT test that you'll *never* hear about from your conventional doctor.

AMAS detects prostate cancer 19 months earlier than PSA test!

When you walk into the doctor's office, they can tell almost anything about your health just by looking at your *blood*. They can detect viral and bacterial infections and monitor your cholesterol levels, blood pressure, and even your liver and heart function.

So why not test your blood for cancer?

Now it's *finally* possible, thanks to a Harvard-trained biochemist and M.D. named Sam Bogoch.

Dr. Bogoch spent 20 years studying how to detect cancer in people's blood. And he developed a blood test called the AMAS, or Anti-Malignin Antibody in Serum. This incredible test is overlooked by conventional medicine even though it has been around for over three decades!

FDA-approved for more than 30 years!

The AMAS test first received FDA approval in 1977. And for the next 17 years the test went through a rigorous clinical study in 4,278 patients that proved its effectiveness. Today the AMAS test is possibly the MOST ACCURATE WAY to test the human body for *any type of cancer*.

Here's how it works: The AMAS test analyzes a blood sample for *anti-malignin antibodies*. Your body naturally produces these in response to cancer cells — any kind of cancer cells.

The best part about the AMAS test is that it detects cancer anywhere in your body UP TO 19 MONTHS before any other conventional medical test! Talk about early detection!

This kind of early detection is especially useful for prostate cancer, which, like breast and many other cancers, can take *decades* to develop into a tumor that a doctor can feel manually or detect through a PSA test. By that time, the cancer might already have spread and become far more serious and far more difficult to treat.

Cancer detection that's 95 percent accurate!

The AMAS test is also far more accurate than the PSA test. Remember, the PSA detects *prostate-specific antigen*, which your prostate produces as it grows larger. The PSA test has a cancer specificity of *only 60 percent*.

But the AMAS tests *specifically* for cancer, and has a cancer specificity of *95 percent*.[73] That means there's far less chance that you'll get either a false positive *or* a false negative result. According to Dr. Bogoch's research, the AMAS

---

72 Henderson, Bill (2008) *Cancer-Free (Third Edition)* Booklocker, Inc.

73 McDonagh, E.W. "Detecting Cancer." *Townsend Letter for Doctors and Patients* (February/March, 1996), 108-110.

test is 95 to 99 percent accurate.[74]

Of course, a positive AMAS test result does *not* necessarily mean you have prostate cancer. It indicates you have cancer *somewhere*, but it doesn't tell you *where*. However, with a positive AMAS result, you can start boosting your immune system naturally. You can also have other tests to locate the cancer.

Surprisingly, the AMAS test isn't routinely offered in doctors offices. And that's not because it's too expensive: It costs only $165.

For more information:

To get an AMAS test, call Oncolab Inc. and ask for a free testing kit. You take the kit to the doctor's office for your blood draw, and then your blood is packed in dry ice and sent overnight by FedEx, along with your $165 payment, back to Oncolab for analysis.

Oncolab Inc.
36 The Fenway
Boston, Massachusetts 02215
Toll-free: 1-800-9CA-TEST
Tel: 617-536-0850
Fax: 617-536-0657
Web site: www.oncolabinc.com

If you'd like to read Dr. Ronald Wheeler's entire article, "PSA — A Barometer to Prostate Health or a License to Biopsy," you can find it online at: http://www.ronaldwheeler.com/psa.shtml

---

74 McTaggart, Lynne (1997) *The Cancer Handbook: What's Really Working.* Illinois: Vital Health Publishing. P. 98.

Chapter Eight

Diagnosing Prostate Cancer

The Biggest Problem with "the Gold Standard"— Ultrasound and Biopsy

In conventional medicine, if you have a high PSA, your doctor might do an ultrasound and then a biopsy to determine whether you have prostate cancer. Conventional doctors call these tests the "gold standard" in prostate cancer detection. Sadly, this process is far from being worth its weight in gold!

According to published research, an ultrasound followed by a biopsy has a detection rate of a mere 30 percent.

In other words, if 10 men with suspected prostate cancer underwent an ultrasound and biopsy, only *three prostate cancers* would be discovered. Why the dismal success rate? There are two reasons. You discovered the first and most important reason in the last chapter:

REASON No.1: *Many of these 10 men NEVER had prostate cancer in the first place!*

REASON No. 2 is even MORE disturbing: I'm talking about missed cancers.

Though experts haven't clinically studied the issue of missed cancers, many alternative doctors have long believed that the rate of cancers missed during biopsy is significant. Their belief is based on experience with patients and on simple logic.

You see, biopsies are taken *only* by random jabs of a small needle. But cancer can be hiding ANYWHERE outside the tiny needle "tracks."

An even bigger problem with conventional medicine's "gold standard" for prostate cancer diagnosis is *damage to your prostate*. And the consequences are far more serious.

How prostate biopsies *spread* cancer

A wealth of research suggests that prostate biopsies, like breast cancer biopsies, can "spill" cancer cells and send them spreading throughout your prostate and even your whole body.

In a study at the University of California at San Diego, Dr. Michael Karin found that prostate biopsies *encourage tissue inflammation*, which FEEDS CANCER CELLS! In his study, Dr. Karin examined cancerous mouse prostates *before* and *after* prostate biopsies.

"We have shown that proteins produced by inflammatory cells," says Dr. Karin, *"Are the 'smoking gun' behind prostate cancer metastasis [spreading]."*[75]

Besides spreading prostate cancer, prostate biopsies also INCREASE your risk of infection.

Painful prostate biopsy damages tiny prostate ducts

To understand how a prostate biopsy can damage your prostate, you need to know what happens during the biopsy procedure.

The doctor sticks a device with a needle up through your rectum (not a pleasant experience.)

---

75 Wheeler, Ronald M.D. (1998-2010) "Dangers of Prostate Biopsies." Florida: Diagnostic Center for Disease.

The needle is shot through the thin lining that separates your prostate from your colon, and into the prostate gland. Then your doctor retracts it, bringing out a small sample of your prostate tissue. He or she might do this multiple times. Many patients say it's very painful.

Alternative doctors believe that *every time* a needle enters a patient's prostate, tiny prostate ducts suffer damage, then become covered with scar tissue. This can cause infection and tissue inflammation — a real danger, especially if you're already suffering from prostatitis or BPH![76]

In fact, there are reports of some men suffering infection, ejaculation and impotency problems after prostate biopsies. There are even documented cases of Peyronie's Disease — an awful condition in which a lump causes the patient's penis to bend permanently. I don't know about you, but I wouldn't want to risk getting this deformity for the sake of a dubious test.

The dangers of biopsy are all the more tragic when you realize that it's now possible to detect prostate cancer WITHOUT a risky needle biopsy.

Now available: "The "Ultimate Prostate Scan" — with NO needle!

Finally doctors can use cutting-edge technology to detect a prostate tumor *without a biopsy*. What's more, they can detect the tumor with such accuracy that they can tell whether it's *localized* — i.e., it's within your prostate — or whether it's spread to surrounding tissue!

Best of all, this high-tech test is safe and non-invasive. It's called Magnetic Resonance Spectroscopy (MRS).

The MR spectroscopy uses HIGHER magnetic fields than a traditional MRI does. These fields reveal the chemical makeup of a tissue mass or tumor. The radiologist usually can tell whether it's cancerous with the MR spectroscopy alone, without a biopsy.

"*As I like to tell my patients,*" writes Dr. Wheeler in his article "Revolutionary Prostate Cancer Diagnostic Scan Avoids Biopsies," "*the difference in scan technique is all about the 'S'. To restate, the 'S' stands for Spectroscopy, or the evaluation of cellular metabolic by-products or metabolites, including Citrate, Choline, Creatine, and Polyamines. The pattern of presentation, including ratios of the component metabolites, yields a 'fingerprint' or cellular identity that predicts normalcy or lack of normalcy consistent with cancer.*"[77]

There is *no other known test* that can determine the chemical makeup of a tissue mass or tumor — not even the Positron Emitting Tomography (PET) scan! In fact, the PET scan often can't reveal whether the prostate tumor is localized or has spread.

So it's no surprise that Dr. Wheeler calls the MRS the most "*sensitive and specific diagnostic test available*" and the "*Ultimate Prostate Scan.*" And he's not the only one raving about this new technology.

The Chairman of Urology and Surgery at Sloan-Kettering, Peter Scardino, M.D., calls the MRS "the greatest diagnostic test that we have ever had for prostate cancer."[78]

What happens during an MR Spectroscopy test

To have an MRS test, you'll first put on a hospital gown. Then you'll lie on your back on a moveable examination table. The table slides into a large tube surrounded by a circular magnet that takes the magnetic images of your prostate. Your head will be outside the machine.

---

[76] Wheeler, Ronald M.D. (1998-2010) "Dangers of Prostate Biopsies." Florida: Diagnostic Center for Disease.

[77] Wheeler, Ronald M.D. (1998-2010) "Revolutionary Prostate Cancer Diagnostic Scan Avoids Biopsies." Florida: Diagnostic Center for Disease. Reprinted with permission.

[78] Wheeler, Ronald M.D. (1998-2010) "Revolutionary Prostate Cancer Diagnostic Scan Avoids Biopsies." Florida: Diagnostic Center for Disease. Reprinted with permission.

Before the images are taken, a technician will perform a basic digital rectal exam and determine where to place a tiny rectal probe that helps capture the images. The test lasts about 45 minutes to an hour.

MR Spectroscopies are available at diagnostic centers nationwide, including Dr. Wheeler's center (see the *"For more information"* section at the end of this chapter). An MRS costs about $2,000. Your insurance might cover it depending on your situation. If your doctor orders the MRS, your chances of getting coverage are much better.

The biggest mistake doctors make with the digital rectal exam

How frequently should you get a digital rectal exam? Many doctors recommend that all men over 50 get them once a year (starting at 45 if you're at high risk for prostate cancer).

If you're having prostate symptoms such as urinary frequency or urgency, once a year might not be often enough; you might want to have this exam every six months.

You should also have it if you test positive on the AMAS test or you have a PSA above four. If your PSA is high, you should also ask your doctor to do a repeat PSA screening.

BUT PLEASE REMEMBER THIS: Any time your doctor does a PSA test, make sure he *always* does it BEFORE your digital rectal exam. A digital exam can *raise* your PSA — but many doctors don't tell their patients this!

Are you in danger of advanced prostate cancer? A simple new blood test can tell you

If an MR Spectroscopy or biopsy shows that you have prostate cancer, the next question is *"How serious is it?"*

Unfortunately, if your cancer is in the early stages and is still confined to your prostate, it's very difficult for doctors to know *if* and *when* the cancer will grow and spread. But there's a brand-new test that can help.

This simple blood test can tell you whether your prostate cancer is inclined to grow, spread and become advanced. The test is for *simple Insulin-like growth factor-1* or *IGF-1*. This is a natural compound found in your body. But in some men it's "unbound," which means the compound isn't bound to a protein. That's bad news.

Brand-new research from Harvard Medical School suggests that unbound IGF-1 is a potent stimulator of prostate cancer cell growth.[79]

In a study of 1,064 men, researchers found that those with the *highest* levels of IGF-1 had a FIVE TIMES greater danger of developing advanced prostate cancer than men with the *lowest* levels.

They found that IGF-1 not only *stimulates tumor growth*, but might also promote *metastasis* (spreading). Most important, the Harvard researchers concluded that testing for IGF-1 might *"predict the risk of advanced stage prostate cancer years before the cancer is actually diagnosed."*

Though your doctor probably isn't familiar with the IGF-1 test, it's a simple blood test that any doctor's office should be able to do on request. If you have early prostate cancer and you can't get the test from your doctor, go to any diagnostic lab near you and get it on your own.

---

79 Chan, June M., et al. Insulin-like growth factor-1 (IGF-1) and IGF binding protein-3 as predictors of advanced-stage prostate cancer. *Journal of the National Cancer Institute*, Vol. 94, July 17, 2002, pp. 1099-1106

Chan, June M. Insulin-like growth factor-1 (IGF-1) and IGF binding protein-3 as predictors of advanced- stage prostate cancer. *Journal of the National Cancer Institute*, Vol. 94, December 18, 2002, pp. 1893-94

For more information:

You can watch a video explanation of an MR Spectroscopy at this Web site:
http://mrisusa.com/

If you'd like to read more of Dr. Ronald Wheeler's article, "Revolutionary Prostate Cancer Diagnostic Scan Avoids Biopsies," you can find it on the Web:
http://mrisusa.com/articles_mris_avoids_biopsies.asp

Ronald Wheeler, M.D.
Diagnostic Center for Disease
1250 South Tamiami Trail, Suite 101 N
Sarasota, FL 34239
Tel: 941-957-0007
Toll-free: 877-766-8400
Fax: 941-957-1033
E-mail: staff@mrisusa.com
Web site: http://www.ronaldwheeler.com/

Chapter Nine

The Hidden Dangers of Conventional Prostate Cancer Treatments

The Truth about Prostatectomy, Radiation and Hormone Therapy...

Conventional medicine's <u>number one</u> treatment for localized prostate cancer (cancer in the prostate gland only) is *radical prostatectomy*, or surgical removal of the entire prostate gland. Most urologists will tell you that radical prostatectomy is a "curative" for localized prostate cancer.

In fact, in a recent survey of urologists, *90 percent* recommended a radical prostatectomy for men with early-stage prostate cancer (specifically, 65-year-old men with PSAs under 10 ng/ml).[80]

But before you let a doctor cut out your prostate, there are some very important medical facts you *must know*.

Prostatectomy increases your chance of survival by ONLY 23 PERCENT!

There's *very little proof* that getting a radical prostatectomy improves your chances of surviving prostate cancer, much less that it *cures* the disease.

A study published in the *Journal of the National Cancer Institute* in 2000 revealed that men who underwent prostate surgery survived their prostate cancers at a rate only *23 percent higher* than the rate for men who did ABSOLUTELY NOTHING![81]

Leading prostate expert Dr. Ronald Wheeler agrees:

"If 10 men with prostate cancer are lined up and evaluated, doctors cannot predict accurately who will be cured and who will fail [with conventional treatment] regardless of who presents with the best disease characteristics.

"Equally unsettling is that all 10 men must receive the most aggressive and traumatic treatment [radical prostatectomy] to yield a 60-70 percent success rate at 5 years, regardless of the choice of Operating Physician or Medical Center selected for the surgery.

"10-year data is another story of limited success and will never be as good as the number of successes at 5 years. In effect, regardless of our surgical skill, the outcome from major surgery is reduced to a guessing game where the outcome always remains in question." (From *Men at Risk, a Rush to Judgment* by Dr. Ronald Wheeler.)[82]

In other words, for many men with prostate cancer it comes back even after radical surgery! What are your chances of suffering a recurrence? The research is shocking…

After a prostatectomy, up to 60 percent of cancers return!

In his book, Dr. Wheeler reports on shocking

---

[80] Wheeler, Ronald M.D. (1998-2010) "Men at Risk, a Rush to Judgment." Florida: Diagnostic Center for Disease.

[81] Newschaffer, Craig J., et al. Causes of death in elderly prostate cancer patients and in a comparison nonprostate cancer cohort. *Journal of the National Cancer Institute*, Vol. 92, April 19, 2000, pp. 613-21

[82] Wheeler, Ronald M.D. (1998-2010) "Men at Risk, a Rush to Judgment." Florida: Diagnostic Center for Disease. Reprinted with permission.

research suggesting that even 10 years after a radical prostatectomy, you face UP TO A 60 PERCENT CHANCE of prostate cancer coming back![83] That's hardly a cure.

And it may leave you wondering, *how can my prostate cancer come back when I no longer have a prostate?* Prostate cancer returns in tissues NEAR the prostate, or in another part of the body such as the bones. Even though it recurs somewhere else it is still called "prostate cancer" because it started in the prostate.

Why such a dismal success rate for the most common conventional treatment for prostate cancer?

One reason for the failure of prostate removal surgery might be that operating on a cancerous prostate causes cancer cells to leak into your bloodstream, where they can latch onto nearby tissues or even onto other organs such as your colon, liver or lungs. In other words, prostate surgery MAY CAUSE LOCALIZED PROSTATE CANCER *TO SPREAD.*

Research published in *The Lancet* in 1995 indicates a very real danger. Researchers monitored the blood of 14 prostate cancer patients *before* and *after* prostatectomies. The results were shocking.

Before the operations, only three patients had prostate cells in their bloodstreams. But after the prostatectomies, 12 patients had prostate cells in their blood.[84] It's clear that surgery releases prostate cells into the blood stream, and if your prostate is cancerous, some of those cells will be too.

Worse, common side effects can ruin your quality of life

One of the biggest drawbacks of radical prostatectomy is that it can ruin a man's sexual function, bladder control even bowel control.

In an editorial in a 2004 edition of the *Journal of the National Cancer Institute*, leading prostate cancer experts pointed to growing evidence showing the "substantial and long-lasting side effects from prostate cancer treatment."[85]

Worst of all, horrible side effects are happening far more often than you're led to believe.

Researchers at the Fred Hutchinson Cancer Research Center revealed disturbing results of a study of 1,291 men who'd undergone radical prostatectomies.[86] Eighteen or more months after the surgeries, an alarming 59.9 PERCENT complained that they were *impotent* and 38.9 PERCENT said they suffered *urinary incontinence* at least once every single day.

Sadly, according to prostate cancer experts at the University of Texas Medical Center, these side effects often don't improve with time.[87] In the case of impotence, the problem usually gets *worse*.

In the Texas study, five years after radical prostatectomies, an astounding 80 PERCENT of men were *impotent.* Up to 29 PERCENT were wearing diapers for *urinary incontinence* and 20

---

83 Wheeler, Ronald M.D. (1998-2010) "Men at Risk, a Rush to Judgment." Florida: Diagnostic Center for Disease.

84 McTaggart, Lynne (1997) *The Cancer Handbook: What's Really Working.* Illinois: Vital Health Publishing. P. 104.

85 Carlos Bermejo, Alan R. Kristal, Steven B. Zeliadt, Scott Ramsey, Ian M. Thompson Localized Prostate Cancer: Quality of Life Meets Whitmore's Legacy Affiliations of authors: Division of Urology, University of Texas Health Science Center, San Antonio (CB, IMT); Division of Public Health Sciences, Fred Hutchinson Cancer Research Center, Seattle, WA (ARK, SBZ, SR) *JNCI Journal of the National Cancer Institute* 2004 96(18):1348-1349; doi:10.1093/jnci/djh282

86 Stanford JL, Feng Z, Hamilton AS, Gilliland FD, Stephenson RA, Eley JW, Albertsen PC, Harlan LC, Potosky AL. Fred Hutchinson Cancer Research Center, Department of Epidemiology, University of Washington, Seattle 98109-1024, USA. Urinary and sexual function after radical prostatectomy for clinically localized prostate cancer: the Prostate Cancer Outcomes Study. *JAMA.* 2000 Jan 19;283(3):354-60.

87 Carlos Bermejo, Alan R. Kristal, Steven B. Zeliadt, Scott Ramsey, Ian M. Thompson Localized Prostate Cancer: Quality of Life Meets Whitmore's Legacy Affiliations of authors: Division of Urology, University of Texas Health Science Center, San Antonio (CB, IMT); Division of Public Health Sciences, Fred Hutchinson Cancer Research Center, Seattle, WA (ARK, SBZ, SR) *JNCI Journal of the National Cancer Institute* 2004 96(18):1348-1349; doi:10.1093/jnci/djh282

PERCENT suffered <u>regular bowel urgency</u> — the need to urgently or frequently move your bowels.

That's a great deal of suffering to go through after a painful surgery that might not even cure your prostate cancer!

Radiation treatments are no better. Many men who undergo prostate radiation fare *even worse* than those who have surgery! In fact, recent research suggests that radiation INCREASES your chances of dying from prostate cancer.

Prostate radiation increases your danger of dying from prostate cancer by 81 percent!

A study done at the famous Johns Hopkins School of Hygiene and Public Health found that men who underwent radiation therapy had an 81 PERCENT HIGHER DANGER of dying from prostate cancer than men who received *no treatment*.[88]

This is no surprise to health experts who've studied medical radiation for decades. John Cairns, a professor at the Harvard University School of Public Health, believes radiation is *too toxic* to cure cancer.

In *Options: The Alternative Cancer Therapy Book,* author Richard Walters quotes John Cairns as saying, "*The majority of cancers cannot be cured by radiation because the dose of X-rays required to kill all the cancer cells would also kill the patient.*"[89]

One of the dangers of radiation is that it causes cancer, especially prostate cancer.

Radiation is like fertilizer for prostate cancer cells

John Diamond, M.D., and Lee Cowden, M.D., have reported on evidence that radiation can *fuel* the growth of prostate cancer cells. In her book *Outsmart Your Cancer*, Tanya Harter Pierce quotes the two doctors as saying:

"Radiation therapy — implanting radiation seeds in the prostate gland — routinely given for early signs of prostate cancer, can actually hasten the development of that cancer. Prostate cells can double in as little as 1.2 months after radiation treatment, while unradiated prostate cancer cells may take an average of 4 years to double." [90]

Radiation treatments for cancer not only don't improve your chances of surviving prostate cancer, a growing body of clinical data shows that they also cause NEW, SECONDARY CANCERS.

But before I tell you about the alarming research, you need to understand that doctors commonly use two <u>special kinds</u> of radiation treatments for prostate cancer.

Two common radiation treatments for prostate cancer

You can get *radioactive seeds* implanted into your prostate gland in a technique called *brachytherapy*. You can also get *external beam irradiation*. As the name suggests, the radiation comes from an external machine that concentrates radiation onto your prostate gland.

Though these two radiation delivery systems are far more precise than the radiation treatments of 50 years ago, it's still impossible to confine the radiation to your prostate. Surrounding organs and tissues such as your bladder, rectum and testicles are still very much exposed to radiation. And that's why research shows that any radiation to your prostate is dangerous.

---

[88] Barry, Michael J., et al. Outcomes for men with clinically nonmetastatic prostate carcinoma managed with radical prostatectomy, external beam radiotherapy, or expectant management: a retrospective analysis. *Cancer*, Vol. 91, June 15, 2001, pp. 2302-14

[89] Walters, Richard. (1993) *Options: The Alternative Cancer Therapy Book.* Pennsylvania: Paragon Press. P. 103-104.

[90] Harter Pierce, Tanya, M.A., MFCC (2009) *Outsmart Your Cancer (2nd Edition)*. Nevada: Thoughtworks Publishing. P. 339.

Brachytherapy *and* external beam radiation cause new cancers

In a gigantic study published in the journal *Urology* in 2008, researchers at Columbia University and the Mount Sinai Medical Center examined the medical records of 243,082 men who'd received treatment for prostate cancer between 1988 and 2003.[91] They found a "statistically significant" increase in both *bladder* and *rectal* cancer in men who'd received external beam radiotherapy or external beam radiotherapy with brachytherapy.

Researchers concluded that men who'd had external beam radiotherapy had an 88 PERCENT GREATER DANGER of developing bladder cancer and a 26 PERCENT GREATER DANGER of developing rectal cancer, compared with men who'd had the whole prostate removed surgically.

Men who received BOTH external beam radiotherapy and brachytherapy ran an 85 PERCENT GREATER DANGER of bladder cancer and a 21 PERCENT GREATER DANGER of rectal cancer, compared with men who'd had the whole prostate removed.

Though these numbers are alarming in and of themselves, they're *really* frightening when you realize they could still climb higher. Most research on the dangers of radiation looks at a span of *15 to 20 years between exposure and cancer*. This study was done within as little as *five years*. The number of cancers in these patients could skyrocket over the next decade or two – and it's ALREADY 21 percent greater based on the results as of 2008.

Advanced prostate cancer: The castration "solution"

In advanced prostate cancers, such as Stage D and late Stage C cancers that have spread to other organs and tissues in your body, doctors often recommend a *"Total Androgen Blockade"*. This means blocking testosterone, the male "androgen" hormone, from entering your bloodstream where doctors believe it fuels the growth of prostate cancer.

The hormone therapy that doctors most commonly recommend is an *orchiectomy,* or surgical castration. During the operation, a surgeon removes your testicles (where you make the bulk of your testosterone), but leaves your scrotum and penis intact.

As you can imagine, men suffer many terrible side effects from this painful surgery, including sterility, loss of sexual desire, impotence, intolerable hot flashes, weight gain, brittle bones and even breast enlargement.[92] Not to mention the emotional pain!

And now there's a newer kind of hormone therapy called *"chemical castration."* In this approach, doctors inject or surgically implant drugs to lower or completely block your body's ability to produce testosterone.

Many men are choosing this over surgery. And who can blame them. But sadly, chemical castration's side effects are almost the same as those of regular castration: loss of sexual desire, impotence, loss of muscle mass and strength, intolerable hot flashes, weight gain, brittle bones and personality changes.[93]

Abarelix: "Chemical castration" drug fast-tracked by the FDA, only to be quietly yanked off the market!

One of the chemical castration drugs, Abarelix (Plenaxis), was fast-tracked through the FDA review process in 2001.[94] But in 2005, the maker

---

91 *Urology*. 2008. Quoted on Wascher, Robert A. MD, FACS. (2008) Health Report: Radiation Treatment of Prostate Cancer & Risk of Second Cancers. Dr. Wascher is an oncologic surgeon and the Director of the Division of Surgical Oncology at Newark Beth Israel Medical Center. www.doctorwascher.com

92 WebMd.com

93 Stephan L. Werner, M.D., F.A.C.S. http://www.wmfurology.com/pcahormone.htm.

94 Article, Urological Sciences Research Foundation web repository, January 25, 2001. http://www.usrf.org/breakingnews/bn_010125_abarelix.html

abruptly took the drug off the market without any explanation.[95] There are no published reports on Abarelix's dangers, other than some severe allergic reactions. We can only assume the drug's maker knows something the rest of us don't. And usually that's not good news.

Whether these drugs are safe or not, what's most important for you to understand is that neither chemical castration nor surgical castration can cure your prostate cancer!

In fact, doctors — even the American Cancer Society — admit that years down the road, prostate cancer cells become *"hormone-resistant"* and start growing again.[96] At best, these painful, misery-causing procedures only buy you some time.

So what happens when castration — surgical or chemical — fails? Doctors go back to their old standby: *chemotherapy.*

Chemotherapy: ZERO survivors of prostate cancer in clinical study

Chemotherapy has long proven a failure in treating patients with cancers of the breast, lung, colon and prostate. In fact, a comprehensive review of these cancers done at the Heidelberg Tumor Center in Germany found ONLY THREE PERCENT OF ALL PATIENTS got any help from chemotherapy drugs.[97]

Another study here in the USA found chemo *even less effective!* The study, published in the journal *Clinical Oncology* in December, 2004, said chemotherapy *has an average five-year survival rate of barely more than two percent for all cancers.*[98] And for prostate cancer it was 0 PERCENT. That's right, there were NO SURVIVORS WHATSOEVER attributed to chemotherapy.

The study tracked 23,242 patients with prostate cancer who underwent chemotherapy. At the end of five years, not one of the 23,242 men was still alive. Of course, these were likely late-stage cancer patients. Still, it's an astonishing failure.

More research confirms the dismal statistics. It seems that chemotherapy drugs for prostate cancer are *not successful.* Two large, randomized, phase III clinical trials of the chemotherapy drug mitoxantrone in advanced prostate cancer patients between 1996 and 1999 found "no evidence of a survival benefit."[99] However, a third of the patients did experience pain-relief.

Further research on another drug called docetaxel showed that compared with mitoxantrone, median survival time in advanced prostate cancer patients increased by only TWO TO TWO-AND-A-HALF MONTHS.[100]

Some men in this study also experienced pain relief as well as improved bowel and urinary function. Of course, in this study and in the one mentioned earlier, some men suffered the usual sickening side effects, including fever, nausea and vomiting from treatment.

---

95 "Hormone (Androgen Deprivation) Therapy." American Cancer Society. www.cancer.org.

96 Article, Urological Sciences Research Foundation web repository, January 25, 2001. http://www.usrf.org/breakingnews/bn_010125_abarelix.html

97 Diamond, W. John., M.D., W. Lee Cowden, M.D., and Burton Goldberg. *An Alternative Medicine Definitive Guide to Cancer.* Tiburon, California: Future Medicine Publishing, Inc., 1997.

98 Morgan G, Ward R, Barton M. The contribution of cytotoxic chemotherapy to 5-year survival in adult malignancies. *Clin Oncol (R Coll Radiol).* 2004 Dec;16(8):549-60.

99 Tannock IF, et al. Chemotherapy with mitoxantrone plus prednisone or prednisone alone for symptomatic hormone- resistant prostate cancer: A Canadian randomized trial with palliative endpoint. *J Clin Oncol* 14:1756-1764, 1996.
Kantoff PW, et al. Hydrocortisone with or without mitoxantrone in hormone-refractory prostate cancer: results of the Cancer and Leukemia Group B 9182 study. *J Clin Oncol* 17:2506-2513,1999.

100 Petrylak DP, et al. Docetaxel and estramustine compared with mitoxantrone and prednisone for advanced refractory prostate cancer. *N Engl J Med* 351:1513-1520,2004.

Chemotherapy for prostate cancer — patients say, "Why bother?"

The Prostate Cancer Research Institute (PCRI), founded in 1996 by medical oncologists Stephen B. Strum and Mark C. Scholz, with support from the Daniel Freeman Hospital Foundation in Southern California, issued a newsletter in May, 2006, with an article entitled "Chemotherapy for Prostate Cancer — Why Bother?"[101]

The article quotes an 11-year advanced prostate cancer survivor and patient advocate who attended a prostate cancer support meeting where people were discussing this research. The man said, *"I speak to guys with advanced disease every day. They read these studies, and they say to me, 'You've gotta be kidding me; if I do chemotherapy I'm going to live 2 to 2 1/2 months longer. Why bother?'"*

His sentiments were echoed in an editorial by leading prostate cancer experts at the University of Texas Medical Center, who publicly asked, *"How many men would accept these risks [of surgery, radiation, chemotherapy] if they knew that often, definitive treatment will not affect the risk of prostate cancer death?"*[102]

I, for one, would not. But I certainly don't want to get sick and die of advanced prostate cancer, either. And that fear of sickness and death is the reason why so many men are willing to listen to their doctors and undergo torturous prostate "treatments." The prevailing attitude is "Do something – ANYTHING!" Even if the treatment is useless.

But it doesn't have to be that way. As you've seen in this Special Report, there are many safe, alternative treatments for prostate cancer. These treatments will NOT leave you impotent and in diapers, suffering from weight gain or breast enlargement, or discovering a second cancer five years down the road.

But how do you choose the one that's right for you? Besides the resources I've suggested in this Special Report, you'll find help in the Bonus Reports you received. Turn to the Report entitled *Your Prostate Cancer Action Plan* for more details.

---

101 Guess, Brad PA-C, Executive Director, PCRI "Chemotherapy for Prostate Cancer: 'Why Bother?'" *PCRI Insights*, May, 2006, vol. 9 no.2

102 Carlos Bermejo, Alan R. Kristal, Steven B. Zeliadt, Scott Ramsey, Ian M. Thompson Localized Prostate Cancer: Quality of Life Meets Whitmore's Legacy Affiliations of authors: Division of Urology, University of Texas Health Science Center, San Antonio (CB, IMT); Division of Public Health Sciences, Fred Hutchinson Cancer Research Center, Seattle, WA (ARK, SBZ, SR) *JNCI Journal of the National Cancer Institute* 2004 96(18):1348-1349; doi:10.1093/jnci/djh282

Chapter Ten
Why So Much Prostate and Breast Cancer?
The Truth about a "Hidden" Epidemic!

An epidemic of cancer is silently ravaging our nation. If you yourself don't suffer from breast cancer or prostate cancer during your lifetime, someone you know or love will.

Too much bad stuff going into our bodies, and not enough good stuff.

The "bad stuff" I'm talking about is the overwhelming number of toxins we get — from chemical pollutants in our food, air and water to the emotional stress in our daily lives.

These toxins sap our immune systems and send our hormones dangerously out of whack. The end result is breast and prostate cancer. Here's why: *Toxins trigger an increase in our estrogen levels.* This acts like FERTILIZER for breast and prostate cancers!

The most dangerous toxins are called *xenoestrogens* ("xeno" means "stranger").

Xenoestrogens are dooming us to cancer (and the government knows it!)

Xenoestrogens are coming from our food, our air, our water and even our medicines. This might be the first you've ever heard of xenoestrogens, but medical researchers have known about them for decades. What's more, they've linked them to breast and prostate cancer for MORE THAN 15 YEARS — even in research by leading government scientists!

Just look at this shocking quote from a study published by scientists at the U.S. Department of Health and Human Services (HHS) 'way back in 1993.

"Experimental evidence reveals that compounds such as some chlorinated organics, polycyclic aromatic hydrocarbons (PAHs), triazine herbicides, and pharmaceuticals affect estrogen production and metabolism and thus function as xenoestrogens. ***Many of these xenoestrogenic compounds also experimentally induce mammary carcinogenesis (breast cancer)...***"[103]

The HHS researchers go on to say that *"most breast cancers"* are caused NOT by a woman's genetic history but by the hormonal changes from the xenoestrogens that toxins in our bodies produce *EVERY SINGLE DAY!*

That bears repeating: **Government scientists have linked the vast majority of breast cancers to environmental toxins, not genetics.**

And here's even more disturbing proof: The rising number of men with *male breast cancer!*

The hidden epidemic of male breast cancer on a leading U.S. military base

Though male breast cancer is still rare in the

---
[103] D L Davis, et al. Office of the Assistant Secretary for Health, Department of Health and Human Services, Washington, DC 20201. Medical hypothesis: xenoestrogens as preventable causes of breast cancer. *Environ Health Perspective* 1993 October; 101(5): 372–377

USA, with fewer than 1,900 cases annually, men who get it often have had high exposure to toxins that produce xenoestrogens.

One of the most shocking stories of male breast cancer comes from the Marine Corps base at Camp Lejeune, North Carolina. AT LEAST 19 MEN who were stationed or who worked at Camp Lejeune have been diagnosed with the disease over the last two years, according to a 2009 article in the *Los Angeles Times*.[104]

These men are among 1,600 former base residents who are *suing the federal government*, saying their cancers and other illnesses were caused by drinking base tap water that the government *knew* was tainted with "chlorinated solvents" as far back as 1980.

If you recall, chlorinated solvents are among the toxins that government researchers *know* to produce cancer-causing xenoestrogens in the human body. The lawsuit suggests a government cover-up that endangered the lives of thousands of men, women and children! The lawsuit is pending.

But it's not just *breast cancer* that's afflicting our brave Marines at Camp Lejeune, either.

Prostate cancer rates, too, are high in these Marines!

One of the "other cancers" the Camp Lejeune men suffer from is prostate cancer.[105] This won't surprise anyone who's researched the development of breast and prostate cancer. You see, we now know that prostate cancer is ALSO caused by toxins that produce *xenoestrogens* and result in dangerous estrogen buildup in men's bodies.

Dr. HingHau Tsang calls this terrible buildup of estrogen "*estrogen dominance.*"[106] A natural health doctor, he's reported on several studies that show that when prostate cells are exposed to estrogen, they grow like crazy and become cancerous.

Other research proves Dr. Tsang's findings.

It includes dozens more studies showing that farm workers with the HIGHEST EXPOSURE to pesticides and herbicides (which create xenoestrogens in the body) here in the USA and other countries suffer the HIGHEST RISK of prostate cancer and infertility.[107]

But most alarming of all is the clinical evidence taken directly from people's breast and prostate tumors.

Send a tumor sample to a toxicologist instead of an oncologist and you'll discover something shocking!

When toxicologists examine tissue samples from cancerous tumors in people's breasts or prostates, they often find *abnormally high* levels of dangerous chemicals.

In his book *Cancer Diagnosis: What to Do Next,* Dr. Burton Goldberg recounts one such story. He explains how a man diagnosed with prostate cancer had a tissue biopsy sent to a toxicologist. The toxicologist found unusually high levels of dangerous chemicals, including arsenic, DDT and chlordane![108]

The research is beyond alarming. But it raises the question: *If chemicals in our air, our water, our food and our medicines are so dangerous, then how come ALL of us don't come down with tumors in our prostates or breasts?*

---

104 Zucchino, David (2009) Camp Lejeune Residents Blame Rare Cancer Cluster on The Water. Los Angeles: *Los Angeles Times*.

105 Byron, Andrea. A Toxic Tale: Water Contamination at Camp Lejeune 1 *Veterans Today* Posted online February 22, 2008.

106 Tsang, HingHau. Dr. Tsang's Crusade on Nutrition. *Newsletter #75 - Estrogen Dominance, Natural Progesterone and Men.*

107 Salinger, Lawrence M. (2005) *Encyclopedia of White-Collar and Corporate Crime, Volume 1*. California: Sage Publications.

108 Diamond, John W. M.D., Cowden, W. Lee M.D., Goldberg, Burton (2000) *Cancer Diagnosis: What to Do Next*. California: AlternativeMedicine.com. P. 15.

After examining years of research, I believe the answer holds the secret not only of *preventing* breast and prostate cancer, but of *curing it* as well.

The simple secret to living free from prostate and breast cancer

What is this astonishingly simple secret? *An ironclad immune system.*

When your immune system is powered up to a high level, your body can rid itself of these xenoestrogens and correct any abnormal hormonal changes they cause *BEFORE* they trigger cancer.

Only when your immune system is weakened by health problems, poor diet, stress and toxins do xenoestrogens get the upper hand and cancer takes root. If you strengthen your immune system, you can help your body defeat breast and prostate cancers *once and for all!*

In the book *Cancer Diagnosis: What to Do Next*, Dr. Wolfgang Kostler, M.D., is quoted as saying that the reason why conventional medicine fails to cure breast cancer is that it focuses solely on *removing* or *shrinking* the tumor, not on *changing* "the cancer-prone environment inside the body." And because of this fateful mistake, the cancer never goes away completely.[109]

For the last 32 years, Dr. Kostler has helped his patients whip breast cancer by supporting their immune systems. This, Dr. Kostler says, is the ONLY way to keep cancer from either growing or returning.[110]

As you've discovered in this Special Report, beating prostate cancer also comes down to *building up your immune system.*

And that's the reason why conventional treatments for breast and prostate cancer fail so many patients: they do *just the opposite.*

I believe it makes absolutely no sense to repeatedly attack breast and prostate cancers with chemotherapy, radiation and drastic surgery. Yet that's exactly what mainstream doctors want *you* to do!

When we were young, most of us had it ingrained in us that we should never question our doctor. Doctors are the *experts.* They *know* what to do. We *must listen.*

That's why so many cancer patients never ask *why* a doctor recommends slicing off a breast, cutting out a prostate, poisoning a tumor with chemo or burning it with radiation — even though these treatments *clearly make cancer patients SICKER and encourage their cancers to SPREAD!*

It's *your* body, and YOU have control!

I strongly urge you to ask your doctor *"why"* when he or she prescribes *any* treatment. The answer you get should be solid and based on *success* with other patients who have your type and stage of prostate cancer. And your doctor should answer any and every question you have. If he or she doesn't, run for the hills!

I'm reminded of a personal story from Timothy Brantley N.D., Ph.D. In his book *The Cure: Heal Your Body, Save Your Life,* Dr. Brantley recalls being a young boy who watched breast and colon cancer overtake his mother.

One day he went with his mom to a doctor's appointment. He was sitting quietly nearby, listening to the M.D. talk, when he felt inspired to ask a question.

"Doctor," he said, "why did Mom get cancer?"

His mother apologized immediately for her outspoken young son. But the future Dr. Brantley turned to her and said, "Well, don't *you* want to know?"

---

[109] Diamond, John W. M.D., Cowden, W. Lee M.D., Goldberg, Burton (2000) *Cancer Diagnosis: What to Do Next.* California: AlternativeMedicine.com P. 199.

[110] McTaggart, Lynne (1997) *The Cancer Handbook: What's Really Working.* Illinois: Vital Health Publishing. P. 196.

That's when the M.D. proclaimed irritatingly, "That's enough questions, young man." The doctor *never* answered any of his questions.

Eventually, Dr. Brantley's mom passed away from cancer. Even more tragic, she spent the final months of her life suffering terribly from the side effects of chemotherapy.

Today, Dr. Brantley and many other alternative doctors understand that treatment for cancer doesn't have to be filled with pain, suffering and loss. You can not only treat your prostate cancer or any other cancer *safely*, you can feel *stronger* and *healthier* during the healing process.

In this Special Report you've seen some of the *best* and *most successful* treatments ever discovered for prostate cancer. I'm not going to tell you any treatment is 100% effective – nothing's even close to being that good – but these treatments are *so effective* that they're slowing, stopping and even *curing* prostate cancer after chemotherapy, radiation and surgery have failed — when doctors shake their heads and tell their patients, *"I'm sorry, it's hopeless."*

I hope that you or your loved ones will never need them, but if you do, I hope this Special Report provides the vital information you need to heal safely and successfully.

As you've seen, you *CAN* prevent, stop, slow and even cure prostate cancer.

I urge you to share the urgent, life-saving information in this Special Report with any relatives or friends who worry about prostate cancer or who are fighting their own battles against this disease.

Wishing you a cancer-free life always,

Lee Euler